T0324751

Attributing Excellence in Medicine

Clio Medica

STUDIES IN THE HISTORY OF MEDICINE AND HEALTH

VOLUME 98

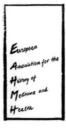

The titles published in this series are listed at *brill.com/clio*

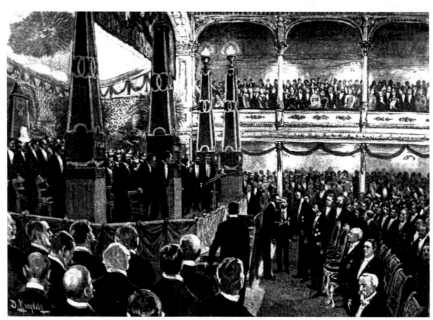

The first Nobel Prize Award Ceremony in 1901. Image provided by the Nobel Foundation. Copyright © The Nobel Foundation.

Attributing Excellence in Medicine

The History of the Nobel Prize

Edited by

Nils Hansson
Thorsten Halling
Heiner Fangerau

BRILL

RODOPI

LEIDEN | BOSTON

Cover illustration: Overview from the Nobel Prize Award Ceremony at the Stockholm Concert Hall, 10 December 2016. Copyright © Nobel Media AB 2016. Photo: Alexander Mahmoud.

The Library of Congress Cataloging-in-Publication Data is available online at http://catalog.loc.gov

Typeface for the Latin, Greek, and Cyrillic scripts: "Brill". See and download: brill.com/brill-typeface.

ISSN 0045-7183
ISBN 978-90-04-39397-4 (hardback)
ISBN 978-90-04-40642-1 (e-book)

Contents

Foreword IX
Jeffrey S. Flier
List of Illustrations XII
Notes on Contributors XIV

Introduction 1
Nils Hansson, Thorsten Halling and Heiner Fangerau

PART 1
The Award and Beyond

1 Commemorating Excellence: The Nobel Prize and the Secular Religion of Science 17
Jacalyn Duffin

2 More Than a Prize: The Creation of the Nobel System 39
Gustav Källstrand

3 Hitler's Boycott: Cultural Politics and the Rhetoric of Neutrality 59
Sven Widmalm

PART 2
Laureates and Nominees

4 From Global Recognition to Global Health: Antimicrobials and the Nobel Prize, 1901–2015 81
Scott H. Podolsky

5 Discovery or Reputation? Jacques Loeb and the Role of Nomination Networks 97
Heiner Fangerau, Thorsten Halling and Nils Hansson

6 Defining 'Cutting-edge' Excellence: Awarding Nobel Prizes (or not) to Surgeons   122
   Nils Hansson, David S. Jones and Thomas Schlich

PART 3
Reverberation and Commercialization

7 John C. Eccles' Conversion and the Meaning of 'Authority'   143
   Fabio De Sio, Nils Hansson and Ulrich Koppitz

8 The Laureate in the Spotlight: Renato Dulbecco and the Public Image of Science   175
   Massimiano Bucchi

9 Nobel Prize Awarded Discoveries and Commercialization: The Role of the Laureates   188
   Katarina Nordqvist and Pauline Mattsson

   Index   207

Foreword

The Nobel Prize is unquestionably the most prestigious award for intellectual achievement and discovery in physiology and medicine. With the early morning announcement of Nobel winners each October, the scientific community and many non-scientists briefly focus attention on biomedicines greatest advances – as judged by the Nobel Assembly. But the impact of Nobel Prizes extend beyond that brief period. As scientists worldwide including many colleagues at Harvard Medical School dream about their future research, many privately imagine themselves winning the Nobel Prize (though they don't like to admit it), providing an additional incentive, if only a remote one, to their discovery efforts.

The Nobel Prize, in addition to serving as the most influential certification of extraordinary achievement, can also be a powerful lens through which to examine many aspects of the scientific enterprise – from the broader role of credit and recognition in science, to scientific discovery as a social enterprise, to the role of science and scientific leaders in contemporary society. Though Nobel Prizes inhabit the extreme end of the prize spectrum, and therefore have many unique attributes, Nobel effects ripple like a force field through the broader ecosystem of science, illuminating general principles of scientific credit and warning of potential future problems in this area.

Why do we care so much about scientific credit? Although Nobel Prizes are the ultimate allocation of credit for discovery, credit serves more broadly as the 'currency of the realm' in academic research. In addition to the pleasure attendant to recognition for your accomplishments, scientific credit is essential to a successful academic scientific career, through effects on faculty positions and institutional resources, grant funding, and obtaining the most highly skilled students and collaborators. Though credit initially flows from scholarly publications and priority, the interplay between publication and credit is complex and imperfect. This imperfection results from many factors; the proliferation of journals with widely varying readership and impact, disparate views of how specific papers have impacted a field, and a host of national, institutional and other biases.

Nobel Prizes occupy the apex of a pyramid of awards and prizes that continue to proliferate. These come in many flavors, and decorate virtually every field and subfield; some recognize specific discoveries, and others recognize career achievements. Each brings value to the scientific community by providing incentives to individual scientists, and by enhancing public respect for the institution of science. Awards and prizes may be initiated by professional or honorary societies, academic institutions, or wealthy benefactors like Alfred Nobel, seeking to link their names and legacies to human accomplishment through awards and prizes that may also empower future research.

Although not the oldest such award, the prestige of the Nobel Prize derives from a number of factors. These include the fame of the eponymous founder, the large size of the prize, its intention to be international in scope, the quality of the selection committee and process, and the glittering royal ceremonies at which the prizes are bestowed. Perhaps most importantly, the prizes (though surely not all of them) have stood the test of time, seen as worthy by the scientific community – both for the choice of discoveries and the specific recipients. Should the quality of this track record wane, new candidates for the most prestigious award might someday emerge, but this is unlikely to occur anytime soon.

In addition to being coveted by scientists for the unique recognition they bestow along with major financial and career benefits, Nobel Prizes bring value to additional parties. Nations and universities see Nobel Prizes as reflecting their communal success and impact, and don't hesitate to market these accolades for parochial benefit. Since most basic academic research is publicly supported, prizes serve the additional role of enhancing public support for research. In these ways, Nobel Prizes fuel the future research enterprise.

The effect of Nobel Prizes on recipients is dramatic. Laureates instantly ascend to a rarified level of public regard, sometimes seen as heroes or heroines worthy of veneration. Doors rapidly open to those laureates seeking such passages. Some become public spokespeople for or interpreters of science, while others opine on subjects – within science or outside it – about which they have no expertise or experience, occasionally to embarrassing effect. Winning a Nobel Prize provides no assurance that laureates' opinions outside the area for which they are recognized are either illuminating or accurate.

The factors influencing the choice of Nobel recipients reflect prevailing scientific attitudes and biases. With passage of time, past choices may come to be seen as forward thinking, conservative, or simply erroneous. Over time, prizes have varied markedly regarding their link to therapies vs basic mechanisms, and may be grouped into broad areas such as infectious mechanisms, techniques that enable and advance many investigations, and genetic mechanisms and manipulations, to name a few.

In the 117 years since the awarding of the first Nobel Prize, much has changed in the world of science and biomedical research. While individual scientists publishing alone or in small groups dominated early research and prizes, many advances today involve large interdisciplinary and multi-laboratory teams.

This creates increasing tension with the current arbitrary rule that a prize can be awarded to no more than three individuals.

As science evolves, so must our approaches to awards and prizes. The Nobel Prize benefits from its venerable traditions, and its guardians are appropriately aware of this. But the flesh and blood human beings who steward this remarkable Prize have an additional responsibility. As approaches to research evolve, they must keep the Nobel Prize vibrant and relevant to future generations. Historians of science, and volumes such as this one, will help ensure that they do.

Jeffrey S. Flier
Dean, Harvard Medical School 2007–2016

Illustrations

Figures

1.1   Number of people honoured with each Nobel Prize in Physiology or Medicine   20

1.2   Number of discoveries honoured with each Nobel Prize in Physiology or Medicine   20

1.3   Focus of Nobel Prizes in Physiology or Medicine, displaying increasing reduction from diseases to organs to cells to molecules   21

1.4   Nobel Prizes in Physiology or Medicine pertaining to the persistent paradigm of 'visualization'   22

1.5   Nobel Prizes in Physiology or Medicine related to persistent paradigm of germ theory, including bacteria, parasites, viruses, and immunity   23

1.6   Nobel Prizes in vitamins and genetics demonstrating clusters   25

1.7   Nobel Prizes in Physiology or Medicine for achievements with therapeutic applications   27

5.1   Nomination(s) for Loeb per year   104

5.2   Nominations by countries   105

7.1   Total number of pages published by John C. Eccles (journals or books)   163

7.2   Yearly production, J.C. Eccles, 1952–1974. Subdivided by major areas   164

7.3   Citations of articles authored by Eccles as senior Non-Nobelist 1952–62 (h-index 53) vs articles by the Nobel lab researcher 1964–74 (h-index 38) vs all citations 1929–75   168

9.1   h-index and highest number of citations for Laureates awarded the Nobel Prize in Physiology or Medicine between 1978 and 2013   193

9.2   (A) While 71% of the Nobel Laureates applied for patents, 29% did not (B) Nobel Laureates who have applied for patents together with only academic co-applicants, (49%), with only industry co-applicants while working for that company (9%), and with both (42%)   195

9.3   Patent applications by Nobel Laureates over time   196

9.4   Total number of publications and industry: Co-publication over time   198

9.5   (a) Nobel Laureates involved in starting a company (40%) or not (60%), and (b) Nobel Laureates appointed to a scientific advisory board (55%) or not (45%)   199

Tables

2.1   Reserved and cancelled Nobel Prizes 1914–1938   46

5.1   Reasons for nominating Loeb   106

5.2   Loeb's nominators   107

7.1   Comparison (Eccles 1961) as Non-Nobelist vs (Eccles 1964) as Nobelist review author   166

7.2   Citations of Nobel Laureates by Eccles   167

9.1   Subgrouping of Nobel Prizes in Physiology or Medicine, in 1926 by J.E Johansson and in 2001 by J. Lindsten and N. Ringertz   194

Notes on Contributors

Massimiano Bucchi
is Professor of Science and Technology in Society in Trento and has been visiting professor in Asia, Europe, North America and Oceania. His book on the Nobel Prize, published in Italian and Finnish, is forthcoming in English (MIT Press). He is the editor of the international peer reviewed journal *Public Understanding of Science.*

Fabio De Sio
PhD, is researcher in the Department for the History, Theory and Ethics of Medicine at the Heinrich-Heine-University of Duesseldorf. He works on the history of the Neurosciences and of research on marine organisms.

Jacalyn Duffin
is a hematologist and historian who held the Hannah Chair of the History of Medicine at Queen's University from 1988 to 2017. Her research focuses on disease, technology, religion, and health policy.

Heiner Fangerau
Prof. Dr, is Head and Director of the Department for the History, Theory and Ethics of Medicine at the Heinrich-Heine-University of Duesseldorf. He works on the history of medicine and the sciences, with a special interest in the development of medical knowledge and medical diagnostics in the 19th and 20th centuries.

Thorsten Halling
MA, is research fellow in the Department for the History, Theory and Ethics of Medicine at the Heinrich-Heine-University of Duesseldorf. His research interests include the culture of remembrance in the history of science, historical network analysis, Nobel Prize history and contacts in medicine and the sciences during the Cold War.

Nils Hansson
PhD, is an associate professor in the Department for the History, Theory and Ethics of Medicine at the Heinrich-Heine-University of Duesseldorf. His scholarly interests include the enactment of excellence in medicine and the history of medicine and the sciences in the Baltic Sea region. He recently co-edited the

volume 'Explorations in Baltic Medical History, 1850–2015', Rochester Studies in Medical History (2019).

David S. Jones

MD, PhD, is the Ackerman Professor of the Culture of Medicine at Harvard University. He has studied the history of health inequities, medical decision making, and cardiac surgery in both the United States and India.

Gustav Källstrand

PhD, is Chief Editor of Science and Programs at the Nobel Prize Museum in Stockholm. He works on the cultural history of science, with a special interest in the history of the Nobel Prize. Currently, he is working on a history of the Nobel Foundation and in an ERC-funded project on patents as scientific information.

Ulrich Koppitz

cares for library and John Eccles Archive in the Department for the History, Theory and Ethics of Medicine at the Heinrich-Heine-University of Duesseldorf. Research interests include bibliometrics, history of public health and environmental history.

Pauline Mattsson

PhD, is assistant senior lecturer at Lund University. She is an economist and engineer by training and has had research positions at the Karolinska Institute, MIT, and WZB-Berlin. Her research is focused on topics related to knowledge transfer, the sociology of science, innovation and research policy.

Katarina Nordqvist

PhD, associate Professor, is Senior Advisor at Formas, a government research council for sustainable development in Sweden. She has a focus on research and innovation policy. Previously, she was Director of Research at the Nobel Museum and Secretary at the Nobel Foundation Program Committee.

Scott Podolsky

is a Professor of Global Health and Social Medicine at Harvard Medical School, and Director of the Center for the History of Medicine at the Francis A. Countway Library of Medicine. His works on the history of antimicrobial therapeutics include his books, Pneumonia before Antibiotics: Therapeutic Evolution and Evaluation in Twentieth-Century America (2006) and The Antibiotic Era:

Reform, Resistance, and the Pursuit of a Rational Therapeutics (2015), both published by Johns Hopkins University Press.

Thomas Schlich

MD, Dr habil., is James McGill Professor in the History of Medicine, McGill University, Dept. Social Studies of Medicine. His research interests include the history of modern medicine and science (18th-21st centuries). He is currently working on a history of modern surgery, 1800–1914.

Sven Widmalm

is Professor of History of Science and Ideas at Uppsala University. His research focusses on science and politics, including policy, from the 18th century onwards.

Introduction

Nils Hansson, Thorsten Halling and Heiner Fangerau

Yet Another Book on the Nobel Prize?

In his will of 1895, the Swedish engineer, inventor, and entrepreneur Alfred Nobel (1833–1896) laid the foundation for five prizes in physics, chemistry, physiology or medicine, literature, and peace to be given to those who had 'conferred the greatest benefit to mankind'. Today, the Nobel Prize is considered the most prestigious award given for intellectual achievement in the world. It is used for ranking universities and underlining the scientific reputation of entire nations. The prize has become synonymous with excellence. However, how is excellence attributed to researchers? One sophistic answer is that who received the prize is clearly prize-worthy. Nobel's selection criterion has puzzled the Nobel committee, the public, and historians of science and medicine for more than a century. One reason is that the notions of the 'greatest benefit to mankind' and that of excellence in science do not necessarily go hand in hand. For example, when medicine is concerned there is no clear-cut relationship between discovery, recognition, and implementation in healthcare, physicians may have done good for many people – or even mankind – and still not be considered for the Nobel Prize. Thus, the various Nobel juries have been anxious to consider the two additional basic criteria mentioned in Nobel's will. These are (1) a ground-breaking *discovery*, which was made (2) in 'the preceding year' (in other words, very recently). Thus, excellence in terms of the Nobel Prize reflects a multi-layered character consisting of features encapsulated in the semantic fields of both novelty and reputation.

Much has already been written about the Nobel Prize. Is there really much more to tell? Given the increasing global significance of the award, it is not surprising that its effects on the scientific community have inspired scholarship by historians of medicine and science. Several books have been published on the Nobel Prizes in physics and chemistry,[1] but the broader history of the Nobel Prize in physiology or medicine has not received as much attention.[2] That said, historians and physicians have indeed shed light on various aspects of this award, ranging from achievements of the laureates,[3] their medical

---

1 Friedman 2001; Zuckerman 1977; Elzinga 2006.
2 Crawford 2002.
3 Bliss 1982; Luttenberger 1992; Stolt 2002; Whitrow 1993; Todes 2014.

specialties,[4] nationalities,[5] gender issues,[6] and political factors surrounding some prizes/laureates,[7] to the public image of the award,[8] histories of specific Nobel Prize years,[9] decades,[10] or overviews of the 20th century.[11]

This book has a different approach. The chapters critically discuss ideas of authority and scientific heroism in general. They also relate to the social organization of the sciences,[12] to priority and creativity in medicine,[13] and major discoveries or even paradigm shifts.[14] Following the lead of historiography on scientific merit,[15] the book considers recognition and reputation not only as inherent qualities of an achievement or a person, but also as the result of a good performance and the process of attribution. More specifically, the book focusses on attributing and staging excellence in medicine in a Nobel Prize context.

At the core of this volume is the idea that excellence is not an unproblematic or self-evident category at all. Rather, it is *attributed* by people to people on different levels. The term attribution insinuates a causal relation between a quality and the subject having this quality. Simultaneously, the term captures 'the interpretative process by which people make judgements about the causes of their own behavior and the behavior of others'.[16] That said, our volume does not take excellence as a reason for being awarded the Nobel Prize for granted. Rather, we wish to shed light on the social dimension of attributing excellence in science and ask why excellence is attributed to some researchers, but withheld from many others? Therefore, this volume – with its particular focus on the history of the Nobel Prize in physiology or medicine – seeks first to historicize the aura surrounding the award (Part 1: The Award and Beyond), to analyze the selection process of the laureates (Part 2: Laureates and Nominees), and to discuss its consequences for individuals and in the public eye (Part 3: Reverberation and Commercialization). Attributing excellence to someone is a performative act. This act, in the context of the Nobel Prize, follows certain

---

4   Lagerkvist 2003; Norrby 2008.
5   Bartholomew 2010; Nielsen and Nielsen 2002.
6   Hedin 2014; Hansson and Fangerau 2018.
7   Crawford 2000; Crawford 1988; Widmalm 1995.
8   Widmalm 2018.
9   Norrby 2013; Norrby 2016.
10   Halling, Fangerau, Hansson 2018.
11   Norrby 2010; Hansson and Halling 2017; Riha 2016, Hansson 2018.
12   Whitley 2000.
13   Merton 1961; Merton 1973.
14   Hollingsworth and Hollingsworth 2000; Jordanova 1995; Woolgar 1976.
15   Jordanova 1995; Woolgar 1976; Reverby and Rosner 2004; Frampton 2016; Münch 2007.
16   https://www.merriam-webster.com/dictionary/attribute (accessed March 1, 2019).

rules and internal logics that can be compared to the staging of a play. Thus, we focus on different levels of the act of attributing excellence according to their visibility. We want to understand the social act of attribution metaphorically as a stage play. Similar to Goffman, who suggested to compare social interaction to drama, we intend to investigate how in the context of the Nobel Prize excellence is attributed depending on the scene. First, we look at the act 'on stage' when the Prize is awarded in a public ceremony; then we go 'behind the scenes' during the selection process and finally, we attend the 'after show party' when laureates, media, and the public celebrate, commemorate, or commodify the prize.[17]

Attributing and Staging Reputation and Recognition

Recognition describes the acknowledgement of a person, an object, or a concept. It has both psychological and normative dimensions.[18] As such, it is a central concept in science and medicine. Scientific theories only become facts when a community recognizes and accepts them. Recognition is closely linked to reputation. Reputation can be defined as the recognition of an ability or the high regard in which someone is held. In his lucid study of the *Intellectual and the Social Organization of Sciences*, Richard Whitley highlights the role that reputation plays in the modern sciences. He defines science as a professional work organization:

> it controls how work is carried out, how it is evaluated and its criteria and procedures govern access to material rewards ... research is oriented to collective goals and purposes through the pursuit of public scientific reputations among a group of colleague competitors.[19]

Long before Whitley, Ludwik Fleck coined the term 'thought collective' to describe this personal infrastructure for mutual recognition in science.[20] According to Fleck's theory, scientific facts become real if a group of individuals agrees on the methods of producing facts, on the style of putting these facts forward, and on the acceptance of these facts as an explanatory basis for further work. Implicitly, the element of mutual recognition is omnipresent in Fleck's idea.

---

17   Goffman 1956. See also Bucchi's argumentation in Chap. 8 in this volume.
18   Iser 2013.
19   Whitley 2000, 25.
20   Fleck 1980.

Ex negativo, he explicitly states that research would not be recognized and promoted if it is not of any social importance. No institution would care and above all no young researchers would engage; in short: no public recognition would be granted.[21]

Bruno Latour carried this thought a little further when he argued that science may be represented as a circulatory system. According to Latour, five types of activities need to be studied to understand scientific endeavors: 'instruments, colleagues, allies, public, and finally, what I will call links or knots so as to avoid the historical baggage that comes with the phrase "conceptual content"'.[22] In his circulatory system, Latour uses the term 'autonomization' to characterize 'the way in which a discipline, a profession, a clique, or an invisible college becomes independent and forms its own criteria of evaluation and relevance'.[23] This process of autonomization relies heavily on reputation and recognition. Only ideas that are put forward with the help of recognized methods will gain support; highly reputed experts acquire recognition for their work more easily than others. In that sense, reputation nurtures recognition, if in professional settings recognized authority is based on expertise or power.[24] Both power and expertise are manifestations of social capital (Bourdieu) which ultimately – in the form of reputation – emphasize a scientist's credibility. Reputation – according to the Matthew effect described by Robert Merton (1968) – bears reputation: Recognition is boosted by positions as 'gatekeepers' in international journals and in renowned scientific associations, honorary doctorates, citations, mutual references, or prizes awarded. An award like the Nobel Prize contributes at both ends to reputation and recognition. Wildcards are not selected. It is only given to highly reputed scientists for their collectively recognized research.

Reputation and recognition in their turn rely heavily on publicity or visibility of scientists. Both grow if the scientific community and the public engage with scientific findings. As Latour suggested, scientists need alliances with 'groups that previously wouldn't give one another the time of day'.[25] For example, they need allies, who financially support research and the transfer of knowledge. At this point, the mutual relationship of reputation and recognition in connection to scientific prizes becomes obvious. Prizes do not just honor specific works; they also bring visibility and public attention to certain research fields and the laureates (and those who hand out the prize themselves).

---

21   Fleck 1980, 103.
22   Latour 1999, 99.
23   Latour 1999, 102.
24   Waters 1989.
25   Latour 1999, 103.

To have these effects, prizes need to be staged, performed, and celebrated. Following the ideas of Fleck, Whitley, and Latour, staging and performance are crucial on every level of the production process of knowledge in science. Again according to Latour, the 'mobilization of the world' by researchers 'is a matter of moving toward the world, bringing it to the site of the controversy, keeping it engaged, and making it available for argument'.[26] Not only staging the matter is important but also staging the scientist, the discipline, and those that benefit from science. This idea of mobilization and staging opens the scope for a performative perspective on science in general and on the Nobel Prize in particular. Performances are human actions, which cover inclusively

> a continuum that reaches from the ritualization of animals (including humans) through performances in everyday life – greetings, displays of emotion, family scenes, professional roles, and so on – through to play, sports, theater, dance, ceremonies, rites, and performances of great magnitude.[27]

In the context of this book we understand attributing excellence to someone as the performative act of ascribing prize-worthiness to a person based on the perceived quality of his or her scientific work. The quality is evaluated based on scientific criteria, which are historically contingent, developed in a social process and connected to reputation and recognition. Staging is again understood as the method and process of presenting, organizing, designing, displaying, framing, and contextualizing institutions, disciplines, discoveries, people, and facts. Staging in physiology or medicine starts when experiments are presented in connection to reputation and recognition. Performance and staging gain importance when it comes to choosing and honoring laureates based on their previous works.

Accordingly, we support the hypothesis that there is no way to measure the 'greatest benefit to mankind' or brilliance in science in an objective way. Instead, the whole decision-making process – the awarding of the Prize and the consequences of being awarded; in other words: the attribution of excellence – is an example of performing and staging excellence. Only those who have the necessary reputation are allowed to perform on stage and only those who are in the position to recognize their works are allowed to applaud or to boo. Everybody plays their part, 'and one man in his time plays many parts' (Shakespeare, As You Like It, Act II, Scene VII). The value of roles can be set by

---

26   Latour 1999, 100.
27   Schechner 1988.

various metrics that change over time. Over previous decades, scientometri-cians have referred to impact factors, citations, and Hirsch indices as tools to measure the relevance of a journal or a scholar. Today, a growing number of scientists question their 'myth of objectivity'.[28] There certainly have been (and continue to be) critical remarks regarding scientific prizes as markers of excel-lence.[29] Nevertheless, new awards are established on a regular basis, and the more reputed seem to boost one another.[30] Seen that way, it is not that surpris-ing that the attention around the Nobel Prize is steadily increasing. The staging sceneries have hardly changed over the past 100 years, and they bear strong characteristics of rituals.

Rituals are human actions characterized by standardization, repetition, en-actment, performativity, and symbolic power. They reinforce social structures by linking their standardized and repeated enactment to past and future ac-tions and social orders embodied in these actions.[31] The Nobel Prize ceremony is such a ritual. It follows a standard plan mimicking the courtly culture prac-ticed in royal formalities. At the same time, it is a royal service because the King of Sweden is present awarding the selected scientists with his own hands.

Performances follow standards. If the standards are broken, the social order is disturbed. Errors in the ritual performance do not go unnoticed and some-times cause a public scandal. At the same time, the notion of an infringement of the rules consolidates the ritual and its theatricality: When Jean-Paul Sartre was to be awarded the Nobel Prize in literature in 1964, he declined it in order to cause publicity for his critique of the Nobel institution and its criteria for selecting and awarding excellence in science. He criticized the prize for being reserved 'for authors of the West and oppositionals of the East'.[32] In addition, his 'refusal to accept the Nobel Prize implied a non-acceptance of the conse-cration ritual and its monarchic-academic tradition'.[33] Following an analysis of Burckhard Dücker, Sartre wanted above all to criticize the institution awarding the prize, not so much for the ceremonial rite but rather for the rite of choosing the winner.[34]

The laureate selection process is a ritual that has barely changed since its inception. There are three main steps, each of which stage and perform excel-lence in various forms. First, scholars from around the world are invited by the

---

28   Ramos and Benavente 2017, 1374.
29   Keating 2018.
30   Ma and Uzzi 2018.
31   Stollberg-Rilinger 2013, 9–13.
32   Dücker 2007, 83.
33   Dücker 2007, 83.
34   Dücker 2007, 84.

Nobel Committee to submit proposals; self-nominations are not allowed. Some scholars are entitled to nominate every year, such as previous Nobel laureates and Nobel Assembly members. The Assembly consists of fifty voting members, all of them professors in medicine at the Karolinska Institute. The Assembly also selects the Nobel Committee with around five members; its working body. After the nomination deadline, the Committee invites experts to evaluate the nominees (some of the experts being Committee members). These reports are then discussed within the Committee, which submits its recommendation(s) to the Assembly. Finally, the Assembly chooses the laureate(s) by a majority vote. Some chapters in this book deconstruct this process by analyzing files at the Nobel Prize Archives in Sweden containing Nobel Prize nominations, as well as Nobel committee reports about prize candidates. These reflect the contentious negotiations about scientific recognition.

Thus, this volume discusses social processes in science by asking how excellence has been attributed and staged throughout the 20th century and how particular achievements in medicine have been selected and acknowledged as excellent in their respective fields. More generally the question is what impact prestigious prizes have on various levels of scientific recognition, from the single individual to the state, and how they are interpreted or used in terms of political actions and different forms of capital and prestige.

Introducing the Chapters

All chapters in this volume underline that the Nobel Prize as a phenomenon can be a useful research object for historians in several ways. The period covered by the chapters stretches from the late-19th century to recent years. Even if the prize might not identify discoveries that are of 'the greatest benefit' to humankind, they indicate what was once deemed laudatory at specific moments in time. In the first section of the book entitled *The Award and Beyond,* the initial chapter concerns the commemoration of excellence in a Nobel Prize context. Jacalyn Duffin focuses on the physiology or medicine prize from its inception in 1901. She groups the prizes into clusters of type: first, physiology and diagnostics (visualization, infection, immunology, metabolism, genetics) and second, therapeutics (magic bullets, such as hormones, vitamins, antibiotics, and designer drugs; surgery, and prevention). Her exercise shows that the prizes celebrate incremental steps rather than 'paradigm shifts' (interestingly, a statement that differs from the argument by Nordqvist and Mattsson in Chapter 9 who state that several Prize-awarded discoveries in fact drove paradigm shifts). Beyond the concerns of priority and justification, Duffin discusses further questions, such as how and why the Nobel Prize became the media-infested pinnacle of scientific success. Why do we need to celebrate in this manner at all? Why do we create, tolerate, and celebrate a quasi-religious, ceremonial anointing of individuals, when sociologists, historians, and even scientists themselves make it very clear that every 'discovery' is a complicated endeavor, indebted to many brilliant predecessors from radically different spheres? In addition, what can historians say about the origins, the past, and the psychology of this practice, a practice that touts science as something that it is not?

Gustav Källstrand traces the architecture of the Nobel Foundation during the first four decades of the 20th century. He argues that the Nobel Prize is more than a prize and discusses the role(s) of what he refers to as the 'Nobel system'. By examining how the Nobel Foundation, the prize-awarding institutions and the Nobel Committee for physiology or medicine at the Karolinska Institute dealt with financing buildings and research institutions, Källstrand makes the case that from the outset the Nobel system was a construction where the parts tried to gain autonomy. This argument gained legitimacy by referring to an ideological 'ultimate end' of the Nobel Prize that transcended the awarding of a prize.

If we look beyond the Nobel Foundation and the work in the Nobel committee, it is evident that the prize also prompted political action, as is shown by Sven Widmalm's contribution on Hitler's boycott of the Nobel Prize. Widmalm emphasizes that the status of the Nobel Prize as the foremost international award in science was well established before the First World War and that it embodied the fin-de-siècle dream of progress through friendly competition. He argues that it became vulnerable to political interpretation casting doubt on the ideology that underpinned it; that impartial judgement was impossible in a world rife with political conflict.

The next section *Laureates and Nominees* starts with a contribution by Scott Podolsky. His chapter uses the history of the Nobel Prize for antimicrobials as a window on the history of antimicrobials more broadly over the past century, with certain Prizes serving as exemplars for the treatment of infections for a series of foreseeable futures. These recursive futures themselves have performed important work, helping to mobilize support and funding for particular approaches to infectious diseases. Podolsky then explores the underlying tensions exhibited across such a narrative, and perhaps most fundamentally, the manner in which the awards have been presented and announced to the world.

The history of the Nobel Prize is also a history of changing centers and peripheries in science and medicine. A 2015 contribution in the *Journal of the American Medical Association* raised the question why American scientists outnumber researchers of any other origin who have (thus far) received the Nobel Prize.[35] However, about 100 years ago, the American scientific community viewed with suspicion the fact that no Nobel Prize in physiology or medicine had been awarded to an American during the first decade of the 20th century. At least one American candidate would come to play a larger role in the nomination cycle. Between 1901 and 1924, the physiologist Jacques Loeb was nominated around eighty times for the Nobel Prize, which makes him one of the most often proposed scholars who did not ultimately receive the prize. Loeb's 'nominee career' analyzed in the chapter by Heiner Fangerau, Thorsten Halling, and Nils Hansson.

The final contribution in this section considers the Nobel Prize and surgery. Nils Hansson, David S. Jones, and Thomas Schlich investigate the enactment of excellence by analyzing the original nominations at the Nobel Committee Archive for Physiology or Medicine in Sweden by considering how it plays out in a field that is particularly practice-oriented. The authors underline an emphasis on ideas of genius, scientific heroism, as well as utopian visions of the scientific solution of insurmountable problems, combined with an aspiration of going beyond the traditional limits of medical possibilities (for example, transplant surgery) and analyze how these ideas were used as important arguments in the discussions about Nobel Prizes for surgeons.

Finally, several compendia on the history of medicine use the Nobel Prize in physiology or medicine as a lens for reviewing trends during the last century. For instance, the German medical historian Erwin Ackerknecht argued that the tendencies of 20th century cutting-edge medicine are illustrated by the names of those who received the Nobel Prize.[36] More recent textbooks, such as Jacalyn Duffin's *History of Medicine: A Scandalously Short Introduction* has (at least in some editions) enclosed lists of Nobel laureates to highlight prominent work throughout the 20th century. It is true that some 'key discoveries' in basic and clinical research are represented in the work of the laureates and their research teams, starting with the first prizes at the turn of the century honoring progress in research relating to diphtheria (Emil von Behring, 1901), malaria (Ronald Ross, 1902), and tuberculosis (Robert Koch, 1905). However, medical historians were not the only ones to celebrate Nobel laureates and their achievements. Over the years, the Nobel Prize has evolved to become a well-known symbol of scientific excellence for the general public. Each October (Nobel Prize announcement) and each December (Nobel festivities in Stockholm), the Nobel Prize is widely reported in the international press.

---

35   Naylor and Bell 2015.
36   Ackerknecht 1968.

However, which effects does the prize have for individuals and larger groups of laureates?

The last part of the book takes a closer look at *Reverberation and Commercialization*. Fabio De Sio, Nils Hansson, and Ulrich Koppitz perform a close-cut analysis of one 'Nobel experience', that of the Australian physiologist John Carew Eccles, who received the Nobel Prize in physiology or medicine in 1963. This case study has some similarities with Loeb's Nobel candidacy. While both were supported by acknowledged nominators from several countries, the difference is that Eccles was part of an established 'Nobel network'. The authors emphasize Eccles' relation with the main 'authorities' shaping his scientific and intellectual life, namely, his master Charles S Sherrington (Nobel Prize in 1932) and the pharmacologist Henry H. Dale (Nobel Prize in 1936), the latter being his archenemy in the 1930s-1940s. By the end of the 1950s, Dale had turned into his greatest supporter in the Nobel race. More generally, the case of Eccles provides an interesting example of many relevant issues in the history of medicine, such as center-periphery dialectics (both in a geographical and – to a certain extent – a disciplinary sense); the making of physiology as a science independent from medicine; the relation between epistemology and experiment; and the relation between science, culture, and religion. All these problems are analyzed under the light of how 'authority' is attributed.

The next two chapters highlight more recent trends. Massimiano Bucchi focuses on the 1999 participation of physiology or medicine laureate Renato Dulbecco (1975) in one of the most popular Italian TV-shows: the broadcast of the Sanremo Festival Music Competition. Through an analysis of the show, its media coverage, and an original empirical study of public opinion conducted in its aftermath, the chapter focuses on the implications of the laureate's TV-appearance for the public image of Nobel Prize laureates and of scientists. It also highlights its relationship with some of the dominant popular narratives characterizing public discourse on the Nobel Prize.

Last but not least, Katharina Nordqvist and Pauline Mattsson follow in the footsteps of Alfred Nobel to investigate some relations between commerce and research by looking at the role of the Nobel scientists in the commercialization process (Nobel had himself acquired more than 350 patents). They have gathered and analyzed information from the last 35 years' Nobel Prizes in physiology or medicine, including laureate involvement in industrial collaborations, patent activity, start-ups, and scientific boards. Taking into account changing attitudes towards commercialization (and of universities themselves) over time and some national differences, they suggest that the laureates were deeply involved in commercial activities, with many patent applications, start-up establishments, and other industrial activities.

To return to the initial question: do we really need more books about the Nobel Prize? Already in 1902, Nobel laureate Emil Fischer claimed that more than enough had been written about the award.[37] However, we think that this ultimate accolade in science and medicine still needs re- and deconstruction. The laureates have become symbols of excellence. Excellence in the context of the Nobel Prize, however, is attributed anew every year. Each year behind the curtains, researchers are evaluated in order to be celebrated on stage. The criteria of what is excellent are therefore historically contingent, as chapters in this volume will show. The unifying element in all contributions is attribution based on reputation and recognition. Thus, this book analyzes attributing excellence as a social process. We hope the volume will help the reader to better understand how excellence has been attributed, staged, and defined throughout the 20th century.

We thank Frank Huisman and the anonymous reviewers for their constructive criticism as well as Fabio De Sio and Stefan Mühlhausen, Düsseldorf, for their assistance during the final stages of the book production.

Bibliography

Ackerknecht, E.H. 1968. *A short history of medicine*. New York: Johns Hopkins, University Press.

Bartholomew, J.R. 2010. 'How to Join the Scientific Mainstream: East Asian Scientists and Nobel Prizes'. *East Asian Science, Technology and Medicine* 31: 25–43.

Bliss, M. 1982. *The Discovery of Insulin*. Chicago: University of Chicago Press.

Crawford, E. 1988. 'Internationalism in science as a casualty of the First World War: relations between German and Allied scientists as reflected in nominations for the Nobel prizes in physics and chemistry'. *Social Science Information* 27: 163–201.

Crawford, E. 2000. 'German Scientists and Hitler's Vendetta against the Nobel Prizes'. *Historical Studies in the Physical and Biological Sciences* 31: 37–53.

Crawford, E. (ed.). 2002. *Historical Studies in the Nobel Archives: The Prizes in Science and Medicine*. Tokyo: Universal Academy Press.

Dücker, B. 2007. 'Failure impossible? Handling of rules, mistakes and failure in public rituals of modern western societies'. In *When rituals go wrong: Mistakes, failure, and the dynamics of rituals*, edited by U. Hüsken, 73–98. Leiden: Brill.

Elzinga, A. 2006. *Einstein's Nobel Prize, A Glimpse Behind Closed Doors. The Archival Evidence*. Sagamore Beach (Ma): Science History Publications.

---

37   Källstrand 2012, 7.

Fangerau, H. 2013. 'Evolution of knowledge from a network perspective: recognition as a selective factor in the history of science'. In *Classification and Evolution in Biology, Linguistics and the History of Science. Concepts, Methods, Visualization*, edited by H. Fangerau; H. Geisler; T. Halling; W. Martin, 11–32. Stuttgart: Steiner.

Fleck, L. 1980. *Entstehung und Entwicklung einer wissenschaftlichen Tatsache. Einführung in die Lehre vom Denkstil und Denkkollektiv*. Frankfurt a.M.: Suhrkamp.

Frampton, S. 2016. 'Honour and subsistence: invention, credit and surgery in the nineteenth century'. *British Journal for the History of Science* 49 (4): 561–576.

Friedman, R.M. 2001. *The Politics of Excellence: Behind the Nobel Prize in Science*. New York: Times Books.

Goffman, E. 1956. *The Presentation of Self in Everyday Life*. Edinburgh: University of Edinburgh Social Science Research Centre.

González Ramos, A.M. and Revelles Benavente, B. 2017. 'Excellence in science: a critical affirmative response'. *Cad. Pesqui* 47 (166): 1371–1390.

Halling, T.; Fangerau, H.; Hansson, N. (eds.). 2018. Der Nobelpreis. Konstruktion von Exzellenz zu Beginn des 20. Jahrhunderts. *Berichte zur Wissenschaftsgeschichte* 41 (1) (special issue).

Hansson N. 2018. 'Anmerkungen zur wissenschaftshistorischen Nobelpreisforschung'. *Berichte zur Wissenschaftsgeschichte* 41(1): 7–18.

Hansson, N. and Fangerau, H. 2018. 'Female physicians nominated for the Nobel Prize 1901–50'. *Lancet* 391 (10126): 1157–1158.

Hansson, N. and Halling, T. (eds.). 2017. *It's Dynamite – Der Nobelpreis im Wandel der Zeit*. Göttingen: Cuvillier.

Hedin, M. 2014. 'A Prize for Grumpy Old Men? Reflections on the Lack of Female Nobel Laureates'. *Gender & History* 26 (1): 52–63.

Hollingsworth, R. and Hollingsworth, E.J. 2000. 'Major Discoveries and Biomedical Research Organizations: Perspectives on Interdisciplinarity, Nurturing Leadership, and Integrated Structure and Cultures'. In: *Practising Interdisciplinarity*, edited by P. Weingart and N. Stehr, 215–244. Toronto: University of Toronto Press.

Iser, M. 2013. 'Recognition'. *The Stanford Encyclopedia of Philosophy*. https://plato .stanford.edu/archives/fall2013/entries/recognition/ (accessed March 1, 2019).

Jordanova, L. 1995. 'The social construction of medical knowledge'. *Social History of Medicine* 8 (3): 361–381.

Keating, B. 2018. *Losing the Nobel Prize: A Story of Cosmology, Ambition, and the Perils of Science's Highest Honor*. New York: W.W. Norton & Company.

Lagerkvist, U. 2003. *Pioneers of Microbiology and the Nobel Prize*. River Edge (N.J.): World Scientific.

Luttenberger, F. 1992. 'Arrhenius vs. Ehrlich on Immunochemistry: Decisions about Scientific Progress in the Context of the Nobel Prize'. *Theoretical Medicine* 13: 137–173.

Ma, Y. and Uzii, B. 2018. 'Scientific prize network predicts who pushes the boundaries of science'. *Proceedings of the National Academy of Sciences of the United States of America* 115 (50): 12608–12615.

Merton, R.K. 1961. 'Singletons and Multiples in Scientific Discovery: A Chapter in the Sociology of Science'. *Proceedings of the American Philosophical Society* 105 (5): 470–486.

Merton, R.K. 1973. *The Sociology of Science*. Chicago: Chicago University Press.

Münch, R. 2007. *Die akademische Elite*. Frankfurt a.M.: Suhrkamp.

Naylor, C.D. and Bell, J.I. 2015. 'On the Recognition of Global Excellence in Medical Research'. *JAMA*. 314 (11): 1125–1126.

Nielsen, H. and Nielsen, K. 2002. 'Neighbouring Nobel: A look at the Danish laureates'. In: *Historical Studies in the Nobel Archives: The Prizes in Science and Medicine*, edited by E.T. Crawford, 133–154. Tokyo: Universal Academy Press.

Nobel Media AB. 2014. 'Full text of Alfred Nobel's Will'. https://www.nobelprize.org/alfred_nobel/will/will-full.html (accessed March 1, 2019).

Norrby, E. 2008. 'Nobel Prizes and the emerging virus concept'. *Arch Virol* 153: 1109–1123.

Norrby, E. 2010. *Nobel Prizes and life sciences*. River Edge (N.J.): World Scientific.

Norrby, E. 2013. *Nobel Prizes and Nature's Surprises*. River Edge (N.J.): World Scientific.

Norrby, E. 2016. *Nobel Prizes and Notable Discoveries*. London: World Scientific.

Reverby, S. and Rosner, D. 2004. 'Beyond the Great Doctors' Revisited. A Generation of the New Social History of Medicine'. In *Locating Medical History. The Stories and Their Meaning*, edited by F. Huisman and J.H. Warner, 167–193. Baltimore and London: JHU Press.

Riha, O. 2016. *Meilensteine der Medizin. Wie der Nobelpreis unser Wissen vom Menschen prägt*. Regensburg: Bückle & Böhm.

Schechner, R. 1988. *Performance Theory*. New York, London: Routledge

Stollberg-Rilinger, B. 2013. *Rituale*. Frankfurt a. M.: Campus.

Stolt, C.M. 2002. 'Moniz, lobotomy, and the 1949 Nobel Prize'. In: *Historical Studies in the Nobel Archives: The Prizes in Science and Medicine*, edited by E.T. Crawford, 79–93. Tokyo: Universal Academy Press.

Todes, D.P. 2014. *Ivan Pavlov. A Russian Life in Science*. Oxford: Oxford University Press.

Waters, M. 1989. 'Collegiality, Bureaucratization, and Professionalization: A Weberian Analysis'. *American Journal of Sociology* 94 (5): 945–972.

Whitley, R. 2000. *The intellectual and Social Organization of the Sciences*. Oxford: Oxford University Press.

Whitrow, M. 1993. *Julius Wagner-Jauregg (1857–1940)*. London: Smith-Gordon.

Widmalm, S. 1995. 'Science and Neutrality: The Nobel Prizes of 1919 and Scientific Internationalism in Sweden'. *Minerva* 33 (4): 339–360.

Widmalm, S. (ed.) 2018. Special Issue: The Nobel Prizes and the Public Image of Science. *Public understanding of science* 27(4).

Woolgar, S.W. 1976. 'Writing an Intellectual History of Scientific Development: The Use of Discovery Accounts'. *Social Studies of Science* 6: 395–422.

Zuckerman, H. 1977. *Scientific Elite. Nobel Laureates in the United States.* London: MacMillan.

PART 1

The Award and Beyond

∴

Commemorating Excellence: The Nobel Prize and the Secular Religion of Science

Jacalyn Duffin

About twenty years ago, I was frustrated by the way my history colleagues tended to ignore modern medicine, as if it was too boring or complicated for humanists to bother trying to understand. Without some demystification, I thought, the gulf between science and the humanities would grow wider, while mutually beneficial insights remained silo'd, inapplicable, and inaccessible.

As an experiment, I launched a seminar called 'The History of the Nobel Prize – Who Won It? Who Didn't? And Why?', focused mostly on the award in Physiology or Medicine. It seemed a good way to review medical achievements of the twentieth century – discoveries that once *seemed* new and important, whether or not they remain significant now. Resources were not lacking. Dictionaries, books, articles, and an ever-growing number of websites about Nobel laureates were abundant: some devoted to nationality, race, and gender. The Nobel Foundation's increasingly excellent, searchable website with its nomination database also helped. Historians, sociologists, and philosophers had already produced a robust secondary literature, using these resources and the Nobel archives.

The seminar class became a huge adventure. I learned far more from the students than they learned from me. They would choose a single Nobel Prize, research its history, explain their findings to classmates, and write an essay. As a final assignment, having heard their classmates' presentations, they were to write a second essay about a collectivity of prizes, defined by whatever parameter they chose: scientific topic, nationality, gender, etc. Consequently, I've had the privilege of hearing a detailed analysis of almost every Nobel Prize in Physiology or Medicine – sometimes more than once. It was a lot of fun.

During the 2009 semester, a student's grandfather, Willard Boyle, won the Nobel Prize in Physics for his work in digital photography; we watched her family's home movies about the ceremony. We had class visitors who were laureates – or had worked with laureates. Shifts took place in the students' own trajectories. A medievalist went to medical school; others bent on science ended up in history. We noticed themes and clusters of 'What Was Important' at different moments in time. We also observed that controversy tracks almost

© KONINKLIJKE BRILL NV, LEIDEN, 2019 | DOI:10.1163/9789004406421_003 every award, if you scratch it deeply enough. And we began to marvel at the human *need* to venerate – an aspect of prize-giving that has received little attention. Each year the class awarded its own Nobel Prize to the best research presentation of the year; whether they were in agreement with the choice or not, the students applied their new knowledge of award-giving to explain their collective selection.

In the following essay, I will use my adventures with the Nobel seminar to reveal some insights about trends in medical science of the last 120 years. First, I will take a brief look at who and how many people or topics have won. Then, I review the prizes to identify themes in terms of topic and novelty – or 'paradigm shifts'. Chronological clusters of awards signal enthusiasms or new paradigms. Surprisingly to the uninitiated – but not this audience – achievements in medicine, with immediate therapeutic applications, were in the minority. Moreover, some prizes went to achievements that, in retrospect, seem unworthy. But the embarrassing 'errors' are just as telling of ambient priorities as the more durable awards, and they have influenced patterns of subsequent prizes. In closing I will comment briefly on prize-giving and celebration in general with reference to sociology and philosophy of science.

At the outset, I ran into two 'problems' in bringing non-scientist historians to research on Nobels. The Prizes celebrate *discovery*. But the concept of a 'Eureka-like' discovery is unfashionable among historians or philosophers – and with good reason. Every important discovery arises from another. New observations rarely turn out to be as original as they first seem; most are reformulations of old ideas.[1] Moreover, many discoveries emerge simultaneously by different workers in different places. Scientists are all chipping away at the same coalface.

Second, the prizes assign priority to individuals, sometimes undeserved, often contested, and frequently political. Yet – just as historians doubt the originality and singularity of discoveries, they have also become skeptical of celebrating individual actors of the past. Rather, they emphasize external forces that conspired to place a person in position to observe (or proclaim) something seemingly new. Furthermore, critics of histories featuring 'dead white males', on the one hand, or powerful elites, on the other, called for more attention to the ordinary, the obscure, the continuous and the marginal. As sociologists and philosophers of constructivist knowledge show, researchers participate in epistemic communities sharing questions across boundaries.[2] This perspective provoked a relative decline in scientific biography as a form

---

1   Grmek 1981.
2   These rising trends are exemplified by the founding of two journals: *Social Epistemology* in 1986 and *Episteme: a Journal of Individual and Social Epistemology* in 2004.

of scholarly analysis beginning in the late 1960s and early 1970s, despite its immense popularity with the reading public; this decline, labeled the product of
a 'Cold War generation', has been questioned by Thomas Söderqvist, among
others.[3]

The earliest Nobel committees discovered that a single year was insufficient
to establish the significance of an achievement. Discoveries need time to ges-
tate, to prove themselves for utility and durability. Consequently, committees
deviated from the Nobel's will. The first prizes went to work completed much
earlier – and that gap grew. The first medicine prize went to Emil von Behring
for his work on serum therapy from the early 1890s. By 1905, Robert Koch was
recognized for contributions to germ theory more than 20 years earlier.[4]

Soon, committees began to acknowledge the fact that most discoverers did
not work alone. In 1906 and again in 1908, two scientists shared the medicine
prize; by 1934 it was three (Figure 1.1). Since then, the awards can be shared by
up to three people – sometimes collaborators, sometimes rivals. However having reached three individuals, no more were added, and sharing among three
has become a 'rule' or convention. The increase in laureates for each prize over
time reflects rising domination of teamwork, a well-studied phenomenon in
history of science.[5] The number having 'stalled' at three has been a source of
criticism, as if the prize has become 'a charming anachronism' that failed to
keep up with the reality of scientific work. As Figure 1.2 shows, dividing the
prize among individuals also made it possible to recognize achievement in two
different fields; however, no more than two achievements have been recognized
in each year. Posthumous awards are no longer allowed, unless the designated
laureate has the misfortune to die between the decision and the ceremony.
Ralph M. Steinman died three days before the announcement of his 2011 Nobel
in Medicine and Physiology; the committee had been unaware of his death.

The demographic identity of laureates has been thoroughly analyzed by
sociologists Harriet Zuckerman, Elisabeth Crawford, and others.[6] Winners
are not randomly distributed. The majority are white males, from certain institutions in developed nations, participating in elaborate networks. A good
way to be in line for the award is to work with a laureate. The advent of the
searchable database drew greater attention and criticism over the extent of the
demographic skewing that has disadvantaged women, nonwhites, and scientists in the developing world.

---

3   Söderqvist 2007, 13; Nye 2006; Zwart 2008.
4   Haddad 1999.
5   Wuchty, Jones, Uzzi 2007.
6   Lindahl 1992; Crawford 1984; Crawford 2002a; Crawford 2002b; Zuckerman 1967; Zuckerman
    1978; Zuckerman 1992; Zuckerman 1996.

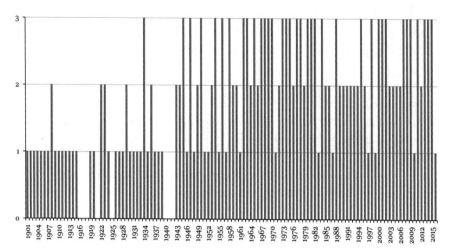

FIGURE 1.1   Number of People Honoured with each Nobel Prize in Physiology or Medicine

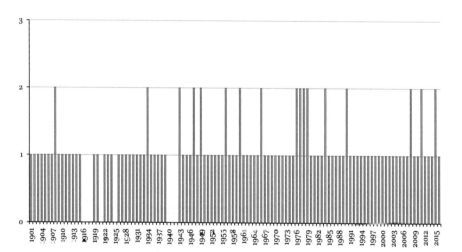

FIGURE 1.2   Number of Discoveries Honoured with each Nobel Prize in Physiology or
            Medicine

The combination of cautions – delay from discovery to award – and pressure to recognize scientists before they die – results in interesting 'push-pull' dynamics that impact choices. A recent article in *JAMA* of 3 October 2016 showed the increasing age of the laureates and the lengthening delay until recognition.[7] One author of this paper, Robert J. Redelmeier is an undergraduate student headed for medical school; he will return later in this paper.

---

7   Redelmeier and Naylor 2016.

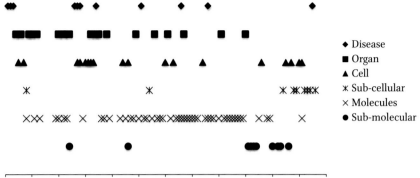

◆ Disease
■ Organ
▲ Cell
✳ Sub-cellular
✕ Molecules
● Sub-molecular

1900 1910 1920 1930 1940 1950 1960 1970 1980 1990 2000 2010 2020

FIGURE 1.3   Focus of Nobel Prizes in Physiology or Medicine, displaying increasing reduction from diseases to organs to cells to molecules

Increasing Reductionism

A big trend in these prizes is toward greater reduction. Figure 1.3 helps to illustrate the change. The medicine prizes that have focused on diseases – that is the whole human organism or even populations – decrease in frequency. Figure 1.3 shows that the 2015 prize on disease is an interesting outlier. Next appear prizes that focus on organs, followed by those focusing on cells, cell components, and finally those that address molecules – be they physiological or pharmacological – or on little bits of molecules, such as ions. Molecular prizes went to familiar names from metabolic physiology – for example, Otto Meyerhof, Otto Warburg, Gerty and Carl Cori, and Hans Krebs. This exercise illustrates two things: first, the overall reductionist trend from 1901 to 2016 and second, perhaps a recent comeback in cell biology – something for us to watch and perhaps explain.

Persistent Paradigms

As a student, I read Thomas Kuhn and even heard him speak in Paris; as a young professor, I learned of and was drawn to the work of Ludwik Fleck.[8] Before launching the Nobel Prize-seminar, I labored under the illusion that Nobel-winning work – almost by definition – *must* be about paradigm shifts. Therefore, a way of analyzing the discoveries would be to uncover what shift each award had effected. But in the end, I realized that surprisingly few of

---

8   Kuhn 1962; Fleck 1979.

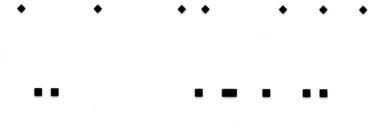

◆ Other ■ Microscopy

1900 1910 1920 1930 1940 1950 1960 1970 1980 1990 2000 2010 2020

FIGURE 1.4   Nobel Prizes in Physiology or Medicine pertaining to the persistent paradigm of 'visualization'

these achievements resulted in major paradigm shifts. Instead, the vast majority merely extended and endorsed intellectual agendas of previous decades. Considerable overlap exists within these themes, and some achievements belong to two or more. Two examples of extended paradigms will illustrate this observation.

The first example is the set of prizes in what I call 'visualization' – achievements dedicated to making the invisible visible (Figure 1.4). One of the great achievements of the nineteenth century was 'anatomoclinical' medicine. Constellations of symptoms were linked to organic lesions that could be detected inside a living patient by tools, such as the stethoscope, pleximeter, microscope, and later X-rays. Rudolf Virchow extended visual pathology microscopically to the cell (he was nominated, but never received the prize). This view still dominates medical thought and disease concepts.[9] Figure 1.4 includes a few Nobel Prizes from medicine and beyond to emphasize the point. In 1901 Wilhelm Conrad Roentgen was awarded the first Nobel Prize in Physics for his 1895 discovery of X-rays. Many creative adaptations were developed quickly, such as fluoroscopy, tomography, and the use of contrast media. Angiography is another X-ray technique was awarded the Nobel Prize in 1949.[10] Without belabouring details other prizes in the realm of visualization include 1906 to Camillo Golgi for the structure of the nervous tissue; 1911 to Allvar Gullstrand for dioptrics of the eye and invention of the slit lamp; 1924 to Willem Einthoven for the electrocardiograph; 1956 to Werner Forssmann, André F. Cournand, and Dickinson W. Richards for cardiac catheterization.

---

9   Kevles 1999.
10   Howell 1995; Risse 1999, 569–618; Stevens 1999, 171–199.

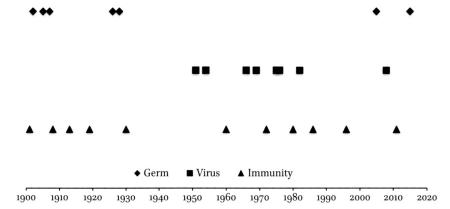

FIGURE 1.5 Nobel Prizes in Physiology or Medicine related to persistent paradigm of germ theory, including bacteria, parasites, viruses, and immunity

Microscopic visualization enters into this pattern too. Originating in the seventeenth century with technical improvements throughout the nineteenth century, microscopy enjoyed several Nobels proclaiming its continued importance into the twentieth century. In 1906, although Paul Ehrlich's Nobel Prize came for his side-chain theory, hematologists remember him for the stains that he devised for *seeing* white blood cells. A cluster of prizes in medicine and chemistry celebrated X-ray crystallography and its applications in 1954 and 1962 to Linus Pauling, Dorothy Hodgkin, Max Perutz, John Kendrew, James Watson and Francis Crick. The latter pair's famous structure-of-DNA achievement relied on the crystallographic images of Rosalind Franklin. Visualization can also be found in prizes for imaging: 1979 to Allan M. Cormack and Godfrey N. Hounsfield for Computerized Axial Tomography (CT-scan) – another extension of X-rays; 1986, to Ernst Ruska, Gerd Binnig and Heinrich Rohrer (Physics) for electron and scanning-tunnel microscopy; and 2003, to Paul C. Lauterbur and Peter Mansfield for Magnetic Resonance Imaging. The 2003 prize also evokes other Nobel Prizes in Chemistry and Physics for nuclear magnetic resonance in general.

Without diminishing the brilliance of these achievements, the medical paradigm served by these visualizing technologies was not new to the twentieth century. Rather they proclaim its wide acceptance by the scientific community and the general public: diseases are of the body and its components – anatomy, organs, cells, and molecules: doctors should be able to 'see' things that patients cannot. The celebrated contributions were Kuhnian 'normal science' refining technologies and possibilities within the paradigm.

The second example of prizes that serve a paradigm originating well before the twentieth century are those predicated on germ theory (Figure 1.5). With origins in the sixteenth-century writings of Fracastoro, the notion of a specific contagion is said to have been widely accepted by the 1880s. To bacteria, parasites, viruses and prions, we can also add prizes on immunity. The idea that surviving a specific contagious disease could convey passive immunity against future illness is evident in Thucydides' account of the plague of Athens of the fifth century B.C. Since the eighteenth century, *active* immunization had been shown to prevent smallpox. As already mentioned, the first Nobel Prize in physiology or medicine went to von Behring for 'serum therapy' against diphtheria – a dreadful scourge that killed little children by horrific choking; scientists and the general public were well satisfied with this award, which helped to launch the prestige of the new prize.[11] Two early prizes went to malaria (1902 and 1907) and one to typhus (1928), while the precipitous prize in 1926 to Johannes Fibiger for his soon-to-be-discredited work on the infectious cause of cancer. Far from waning, the germ theory paradigm saw the 2008 prize go to the AIDS virus. The 2005 prize given to the bacterial cause of peptic ulcer disease, pulled that disease concept out of twentieth-century psychoanalysis and plunked it squarely in nineteenth-century germ theory. Prizes on vaccines and other immunological achievements also stem from concepts originating in germ theory or earlier.

Even as they provide a fuller understanding of self-defence, viruses, prions, and many previously unknown pathogens, the numerous Nobel Prizes in the realm of infectious causes of disease and immunity reflect the persistence of an old paradigm.

Clusters and New Paradigms?

In contrast to the marked persistence of old paradigms, a few clusters of awards allow us to consider the possibility of new paradigms. Many different clusters can be identified, but again two examples will illustrate the point; both have qualitative roots in antiquity.

The first example is vitamins. With hormones they can be thought of as early 'Magic Bullets', although the vitamin prizes were more for physiological understanding of metabolism than for therapeutics. The phrase 'magic bullet' was used by Ehrlich as he tested dyes, hoping to find one that would magically target and kill bacteria (bullet) without also killing the host (magic).

As the ancient physiological explanations of body function were being transformed into precise chemical reactions, scientists turned to diet. After all, Hippocrates had understood the importance of diet in health and disease.

---

11   Luttenberger 1996.

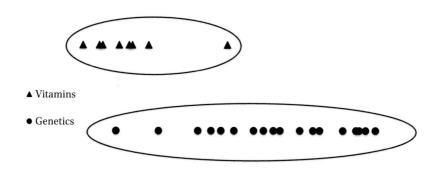

FIGURE 1.6   Nobel Prizes in Vitamins and Genetics Demonstrating Clusters

Furthermore, in the 1740s British naval officer James Lind had shown the value of citrus juice in preventing scurvy.[12] Dismantling and analysis of foodstuffs would further explain how the body keeps itself alive and well maintained.

Reductionist, molecular, and laden with therapeutic promise, the tight cluster of vitamin prizes in medicine and also chemistry – for discovery, isolation, elaboration – suggests a new paradigm (Figure 1.6). The word vitamin(e) was coined by Casimir Funk around 1912 to express the idea that tiny components of food (*amines*) were essential to healthy life (*vita*). Christiaan Eijkman found that brown rice prevented 'beri beri' that afflicted eaters of polished rice. Vitamins meant that several other diseases – scurvy, pellagra, rickets, kwashiorkor, or sprue – might be owing to as-yet-unidentified dietary deficiencies; they were previously considered infectious because they arose in localized outbreaks. They shifted to metabolic.

The second example of a possible new paradigm is molecular genetics. Hereditarian views of health and disease also go back to antiquity. Modern genetics transformed and reduced the ancient, descriptive notions of heredity, identity, and susceptibility into precise chemical formulae. Mirko Grmek referred to it as the third revolution in concepts of life and disease – a new paradigm – for its total reliance on molecules and data.[13] More Nobel Prizes have been awarded in this domain than in any other, particularly in the last fifty years (Figure 1.6).[14] Around 1900, a priority dispute over the notion of inheritance of

---

12   Bartos 2015; Lind 1753.
13   Grmek 2001; Grmek 1999; Burke 2012, 264.
14   Keller 2000.

independent characteristics led to the appreciation of the earlier observations of Gregor Mendel.[15] A century later, the Human Genome Project was set to report on the entire genetic code (completed 2003).[16] Between these two (as yet) *non*-Nobel moments, qualitative ideas were molecularized.[17] Nobel Prizes in Chemistry also recognized work in genetics: recombinant DNA and the invention of the polymerase chain reaction (PCR).

Genetics proved so attractive early in the twentieth century that, in the form of eugenics, it was applied as a kind of scientific benediction to racist policies.[18] It can be no accident that T.H. Morgan received his Nobel for chromosomes in 1933 – the same year that Adolf Hitler was elected to power in Germany. For its scientific status, eugenics was also used in many other countries too, including my own.[19] After 1945, a horrified reaction against eugenics led to funding problems for all genetics research; however, its applications in family planning – including laureate Robert Edwards' work with in vitro fertilization – helped to redeem its status.[20] Having endured the slings and arrows of politically motivated failures and abuses, some genetics laureates became articulate champions for the value of research and public ownership and access to information.[21]

The precise genetic error has now been identified chemically in a wide array of human diseases, such as Tay-Sachs, sickle cell, cystic fibrosis, muscular dystrophy, and several forms of cancer. Even diseases not thought to be hereditary are proving to have genetic correlations – but genetic engineering, or applications remain elusive.[22]

Prizes in Therapeutics

Until this point, the prizes I have discussed are mostly to do with physiology rather than clinical medicine – or therapeutics- achievements that could be applied immediately to health care. They are in the minority, although they make an interesting set of their own. Among them are prizes for antimicrobial

---

15   Carlson 2004, 99–108; Mayr 1982, 710–731; Sapp 1990.
16   Kevles and Hood 1992.
17   Judson 1979; Olby 1974.
18   Proctor 1988.
19   Adams 1990; Kevles 1985; McLaren 1990.
20   Coventry and Pickstone 1999.
21   Ferry and Sulston 2002.
22   Yarborough and Sharp 2009.

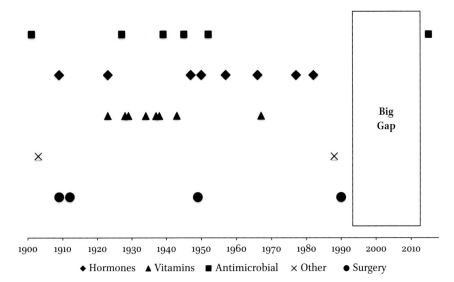

1900   1910   1920   1930   1940   1950   1960   1970   1980   1990   2000   2010

◆ Hormones   ▲ Vitamins   ■ Antimicrobial   ✕ Other   ● Surgery

FIGURE 1.7   Nobel Prizes in Physiology or Medicine for Achievements with Therapeutic
Applications

drugs – more 'magic bullets' (Figure 1.7).[23] This little cluster is intimately connected to the germ theory paradigm, and when it is combined with Nobel Prizes for hormones – and for vitamins, discussed above, they seem to concentrate
at the end of the first half of the twentieth century. Again the 2015 prize stands
out almost as an anomaly, to be addressed below.

Surgery is also part of therapeutics. Despite the tremendous prestige afforded surgeons, few have received the Nobel Prize. Theodor Kocher's 1909 prize
was for his contributions in thyroid surgery and endocrinology. Three years later, Alexis Carrel was honoured for the techniques of vascular anastomosis and
organ grafts. The 1949 award went to Egas Moniz for the now cringe-inducing
'discovery of the therapeutic value of leucotomy [later called lobotomy] in certain psychoses'. Not a surgeon, Moniz was a neurologist, who had promoted
the operation.[24]

If all the prizes for therapeutics are gathered together (Figure 1.7) – vitamins,
antimicrobials, hormones, drugs and operations – two things appear: that
strange outlier of 2015 and a 'big gap' in the recent past. Recent prizes seem
to go to physiology rather than therapeutics. In seeking to explain that gap,

---

23   See Chapter 4 in this volume.
24   See Chapter 6 in this volume.

it is tempting to examine the two therapeutic prizes that immediately preceded its onset. Was there something about the 1988 and 1990 awards that put paid to the competitiveness of future novel therapies? Had all strategies been imagined?

The 1988 prize was a most interesting award honoring three scientists James Black, Gertrude Elion, and George Hitchings. They had used a novel approach to design 'rational derivatives', drugs that would interfere chemically with chemically-defined problems. For example, beta-blockers obstructed internal substances to slow heart rate and lower blood pressure; 6-mercaptopurine interfered with the replication mechanism of cells fooling them into malfunction; allopurinol altered the body's handling of uric acid; cimetidine blocked receptors that triggered stomach acid secretion. Furthermore – like Gerhard Domagk of sulfa fame, all three laureates worked in the private pharmaceutical industry. This prize therefore prompted an appreciation of industrial research in innovation.[25] Using similar concepts during the 'big gap', new rational derivatives were developed to target molecules expressed on tumour cells – the designer drugs – for example, imantinib for leukemia, rituximab for lymphoma, and trastuzumab for breast cancer. None of these brilliant, new entities has yet garnered a Nobel – possibly because the novel *idea* was already lauded back in 1988.

In 1990, surgeon Joseph B. Murray shared the prize with hematologist E. Donnall Thomas for transplantation of kidney and bone marrow, respectively. Like the 1930 award to Landsteiner for blood groups in transfusion – a therapy akin to transplantation – this award was as much for immunology as it was for surgery. Recently surgical innovation trades on the delicate techniques of interventional imaging so that pure surgery begins to shrink and seem obsolete.

Another, possibly better reason for the big gap in therapeutic prizes might be the fact that several earlier prizes in therapeutics – like lobotomy – are among the more embarrassing in Nobel history. Once heralded as triumphs, only to be quickly eclipsed, these awards are especially popular with my seminar students who try to understand how things that seem so wrong now had been laudable not long ago. Did the short-lived reigns of these treatments curb enthusiasm for all therapies in general? Reluctance to recognize treatments may mean that their inventors die before their worth is proven.

---

25   See Chapter 9 in this volume.

Nobel Errors and Interactions?

Sometimes the awards have been premature: notwithstanding the five Nobels given to understanding, using, and controlling malaria, this treatable, preventable disease still claims half a million lives every year. Meanwhile new infectious diseases have emerged, such as Ebola, AIDS, and SARS. Furthermore, the advent of powerful, new antibiotics has provoked more devastating organisms, such as the Methicillin-resistant Staphylococcus aureus (MRSA).

Study of the – from today's perspective – embarrassing prizes, such as lobotomy, prompts speculation on how seemingly unrelated prizes interact one with another. A tentative example can be found in the greatest outlier of all: the 1973 Prize in Medicine and Physiology given to three scientists Nikolaas Tinbergen, Konrad Lorenz and Karl von Frisch for studies of ethology or animal behavior. Only when two of my students gave back-to-back presentations on 1948 and 1973 did I begin to muse about a possible connection. The 1948 Nobel went to Paul Müller, who had developed the insecticide DDT. Used to control typhus during the war, DDT was also expected to serve the World Health Organization's new project to eradicate malaria. But by 1962, DDT had become a source of environmental degradation, decried in Rachel Carson's influential book, *Silent Spring*. DDT endangered species, and by the early 1970s, it was banned in many countries. Hearing two students describe these Nobels in the same class prompted wondering about the influence of social context in decision-making over the awarding of prizes. Did embarrassment over the DDT prize may have had a subtle, redemptive role to play in the 1973 prize, an environmental apology, a way of 'saying sorry' to the birds and the bees? Are other such external influences to be found?

This surprising connection invites speculation on the strange 2015 prize. It recognized work on diseases and on antimicrobials – both topics that had long been ignored with gaps of their own. It also was the first award to go to a Chinese scientist.[26] The parasitic diseases involved were the ancient scourges of elephantiasis, river blindness, and malaria. The laureates had developed drugs – ivemectin and artemisinin – that had a huge impact in reducing mortality and morbidity from these terrible conditions. The science involved in developing the ivermectin from streptomyces bacteria was an extrapolation upon that already awarded Selman Waksman in 1952. The science involved in developing artemisinin relied on granting credibility to a folk remedy derived from plants. Artemisinin came along just as malarial parasites were beginning to

---

26   Hua 2016.

develop resistance to the old-standby treatment, chloroquine. The prize surely was motivated by the epidemiological successes. But I wonder if, in resurrecting long-neglected topics – disease and antimicrobials, the Nobel committee was also lauding *access* to treatments and making a statement about research norms endorsed in 1988: the drugs had originated outside of industry and were without active patents in 2015; Merck had been distributing ivermectin for free. Here again, prizes were talking to each other through social and political currents.

What Does it All Mean? Unsung Heroes, Priority Disputes, and Celebration

The Nobel Prizes are of such prominence that much ado is made about non-winners. Students soon discover that worthy scientists are left out of almost every award: unsung heroes – and unsung achievements. For individuals, the frequently nominated, but never honoured include Émile Roux, Casimir Funk, Sigmund Freud, and Oswald Avery. But other worthy people such as Shibasaburo Kitasato, Nicolai Paulescu, and Rosalind Franklin were never nominated for sadly obvious reasons. Similarly, for discoveries rather than people, the Nobel Prize failed to recognize observations that have saved or prolonged many lives, perhaps because their methods relied on established techniques. For example, water purification methods, global eradication of smallpox by the World Health Organization, Papanicoulou and other cytology smears in the early detection of cancer, pulmonary surfactant in the care of premature infants, safe methods of birth control, polio vaccines, fluid treatments for infantile diarrhea. Similarly some influential theories have been ignored – at least so far: evidence-based medicine, psychoanalysis, and psychiatry in general.

Beyond errors, unsung heroes and overlooked or premature achievements are the ugly priority disputes. Albert Schatz, one of Waksman's graduate students felt wrongly excluded from the award and launched a vigorous protest that probably harmed his reputation and Waksman's too.[27] Possibly the most spectacular of these was Raymond V. Damadian's objection to his exclusion in the 2003 prize for magnetic resonance imaging. He purchased full-page advertisements in the *New York Times* to protest the 'shameful wrong'.[28]

The Nobel Prize contributes to the construction of science as a race toward immutable truths and colossal rewards – as if science were a competition and

---

27   Kingston 2004; Wainwright 1991.
28   Prasad 2007.

discovery a form of archeology, unearthing innovations like potsherds at a dig. This view is held and nurtured by an eager and needy public, expecting new cures and craving immortality. The same view also governs the academic reward system that determines merit by totalling grant funding and enumerating publications in journals of measured influence. Consequently it fosters many kinds of deviance including the aforementioned priority disputes and fraud. But this view does not reflect either the reality of scientific inquiry or the vicissitudes of clinical practice, which are anchored in collaboration, delay, reversal, exceptions, and messiness. False as they may be, competition and the race to truth now define the terrain.

In other words, the prizes can recognize the wrong people and the wrong achievement, and they can generate the wrong message about how science is done. But they are believed.

More than half a century ago, sociologist Robert K. Merton, developed robust theories about scientific discovery, competition, and priority disputes.[29] Citing a 1922 political science paper, he suggested that the vast majority of discoveries are 'multiples' not singletons and they are inevitable. They depend as much (or more) on timing, funding, and intellectual climate as on scientific genius.[30] His insightful essays explain how the norms of science and its reward system generate deviant behavior – the priority disputes and fraud. Web of Science shows that references to Merton in the scientific literature persist and reached more than 700 in 2018.

Intended to be apolitical, the prize is riven with politics and sometimes it spawns interesting, defensive rhetoric.[31] A more pragmatic view of the history of discovery was suggested by Canadian Augustine Brannigan who pointed out that beyond the high-octane realm of historians and philosophers of science, most people are untroubled by erudite reservations over discovery, discoverers, and how science works. Whether or not *scholars* think of discoveries as 'real', the general public well understands the term. Brannigan therefore suggested that credit – priority – rightly belongs to the one who convinces the world, as much, if not more than to the person who made the observation first.[32] If Nobel scientists had not 'convinced the world' before their awards, the Prize certainly completes the job for them afterwards. The awards end up convincing and promoting in a host of other domains, including

---

29   Merton 1973, 286–324; 352–364.
30   Ogburn and Thomas 1922.
31   Sven Widmalm discusses this topic in Chapter 3 in this volume.
32   Brannigan 1981, 50–62, 70–78.

marketing – of universities, institutes and industry too.[33] In preparing this essay, I stumbled on a whacky example inviting 'internauts' to invent and purchase their own Nobel.[34]

The Need to Create Prizes

The prestige of the Nobel Prize reifies the achievement as a significant 'milestone' of medical 'progress'. It turns laureates into heroes and constructs a scientific 'elite', a pantheon, interconnected and genealogical. Many Nobel achievements are difficult if not impossible to understand for the average person. But the prize lends *unquestioned* prestige and draws public attention. Even if the discoveries are obscure, laureates are venerated with awe. Like Olympic athletes, their productivity is compared one to another;[35] a sperm bank once tried unsuccessfully to immortalize (and capitalize on) their genius.[36]

Much sought after as speakers, laureates find themselves expatiating on topics for which they have no expertise, including philosophy and politics. One of the most influential such works was *What is Life?* (1945) by physics laureate Erwin Schrödinger. Other examples include meditative books by Alexis Carrel, Jacques Monod, François Jacob, Peter Medawar, Roger Sperry, and Eric Kandel. I've often thought it would be fun to run a course on these works; at the least, we need a doctoral dissertation on them. Are the laureates goaded into these writings? Do they accept that the Prize confers a duty to display multi-talented and multi-faceted insights on the state of the world? Their opinions enjoy wide distribution as if they ought to exert value-added influence over those of ordinary mortals. For example, in 1992 an appeal for peace in Croatia was signed by 104 Nobel laureates and printed in the *New York Times*.[37] Surely war will end when Nobel laureates demand it.

Beyond philosophy and prophecy, laureates are venerated like holy saints and martyrs – as if science had replaced religion, to give people something or someone to worship. The book *Science is a Sacred Cow* first appeared in 1950. At the time, its chemist author, Anthony Standen, was complaining about unquestioning dogma that had crept into the techniques of science *educators* – not about science *per se*. It's lead, however, together with my experience

---

33   See Chapter 9 in this volume.
34   http://krboerup.wixsite.com/yournobelprize (accessed January 10, 2019).
35   Kantha 1995.
36   Plotz 2005.
37   American Initiative for Croatia 1992, A14.

working on science in medical miracles in the Vatican Archives meant that the similarly reverential religious language often applied to the Nobel laureates leaps out. Many world religions, beyond various Christian denominations, venerate once-living saints, prophets, deities, heroes, martyrs, and their wonderous deeds.

Examples of these parallels are easy to find. Marie Curie was a 'martyr' to her science. Many laureates, like saintly heroes, overcome adversity – disease, loneliness, and political oppression. The Oscar-winning film *A Beautiful Mind* is based on the difficult life of economist John Nash. The author of a 2016 article contends that Jews garnered Nobel Prizes because of their struggles against adversity, including the Holocaust, enhancing their ability to achieve; he suggests that their exodus from Nazi Europe brought the balance of intellectual power to America.[38] In a book on *Heroes and Saints*, we find a chapter – not on a laureate – but on Alfred Nobel himself, written in the vein of expiated guilt – guilt over his brother's accidental death, guilt over having given the world a weapon of mass destruction – a protestant saint.[39]

Like John R. Bartlett's biblical proverbs, the aphorisms of Hippocrates, or the sayings of Chairman Mao, the quotations of Nobellists have been gathered for the convenience of speechifying executives, spawning a mini-growth sector in self-published digital books.[40] Again as suggested above, the prizes seem to communicate with each other in heady narratives of redemption and salvation. American George Minot nearly died of severe diabetes first diagnosed 1921 – but he was saved in the nick of time, so the legend goes, by Canadian Fred Branting's discovery of insulin, which rapidly won a Nobel in 1923, so that Minot could go on to win his own Nobel in 1934 for the raw-liver diet cure for pernicious anemia.[41]

More evidence for this connection with religion is to be found in reactions to Nobel laureates whose behavior dishonours the award and themselves. For example, in the 1990s when Alexis Carrel's Nazi sympathies entered political discourse, calls came to rename the streets bearing his name.[42] When D. Carleton Gajdusek was jailed for sexual abuse of children in 1997, his crimes were aggravated by a perceived indignity against the award.[43] Charges of scientific fraud by associates of Nobel laureate David Baltimore attracted enhanced

38   Pratt 2016.
39   Christensen 1997, 85–86.
40   Chityil 2012; Dingle 2012; Pratt 2012.
41   Rogers 2011, 110; Sinclair 2008.
42   Weksler 2004.
43   McCarthy 1997.

media interest.[44] These 'great betrayals' against the sanctity of the Nobel Prize provoke calls for revoking the awards – as if the Nobel prize itself were not a product of human frailty in a given moment.[45]

Sometimes I worry that I might be projecting these connections with religion onto my object of study – because of earlier work; however, I was greatly reassured just two weeks before our Düsseldorf conference, when I received an unsolicited email from Robert Redelmeier, the student who published on the advancing ages of Nobel laureates. I had given a guest lecture about my research on medicine and miracles at his University – and lo and behold, he made the connection all by himself. He wondered if saints might be getting older – just like the Nobel laureates he had studied.[46]

Few people question the sacred entitlement conferred by the prizes. It is the solemnity of this unquestioning practice that is so cleverly satirized in the annual Ig-Nobel awards organized by the magazine *Annals of Improbable Research* and broadcast on American National Public Radio every year since 1991 (Improbable Research).

Yet why should we accept these ancillary determinations? Why does society tolerate, even embrace, the construction of elites and the attendant distortions of scientific practice? Little scholarship addresses why we make prizes at all. Phaleristics – the scholarly study of awards – tends to report in cumulative dictionaries and databases, like encyclopedias of heraldry – documenting the purpose and ranking the prestige and monetary gains. *Critical* phaleristics, so far indulged in mostly by economists and business people, emphasizes secondary gains for the prize creators: elevating their status, motivating workers, bringing social control over winners (happier employees) and political control over the field, raising and skewing its profile.[47] It seems that we have a human 'need' to create heroes, solemnity, and ritual.

In trying to understand the phenomenon of public *acceptance* of prizes beyond the secondary gain for their creators, I have been searching in the literature of psychology, sociology, and philosophy without much success. The closest I can find are studies on 'the human need to compete' – or 'the human need to worship', the former devoted to analysis of war and sport – the latter to studies of religion. Sometimes these 'needs' are viewed as pathological – cravings, 'addictions' – ripe for treatment and elimination. Yet, while the

---

44   Kevles 1998.
45   Judson 2004, 191–243.
46   Personal communication, Robert J. Redelmeier to J. Duffin, e-mail message, 29 October 2016, with permission.
47   Goode 1978; Chan, Frey, Gallus et al. 2014; Frey and Gallus 2015; Frey and Gallus 2017.

Science Citation Index reveals hundreds of references to Merton each year, few scientific articles (sometimes none!) cite philosophers and sociologists who have written with epistemic justifications and refutations of these needs, the human compulsion to compete, to worship, to venerate: Karl Marx, Émile Durkheim, Max Weber, Jerome Gellman, Pierre Bourdieu.

Perhaps in analogous form both 'needs' (to compete and to worship) are addressed by not the giving, but by the *creation* and the *consumption* of prizes. There is a huge children's literature on bible stories – and we find a bright reflection of the same for science and Nobel laureates – delivering inspiration in narratives of overcoming obstacles and conquering problems. These are optimistic stories for a world that is skeptical of saints and unbelieving in God, and ready for the secular religion of science.

Bibliography

Adams, M.B. 1990. *The Wellborn Science: Eugenics in Germany, France, Brazil, and Russia*. New York: Oxford University Press.

American Initiative for Croatia. 1992. 'An appeal for by 104 Nobel laureates for peace in Croatia'. *New York Times*, 14 January.

Bartos, H. 2015. *Philosophy and Dietetics in the Hippocratic On regimen: a Delicate Balance of Health*. Leiden and Boston: Brill.

Brannigan, A. 1981. *The Social Basis of Scientific Discoveries*. Cambridge: Cambridge University Press.

Burke, P. 2012. *Social History of Knowledge*. Cambridge: Polity.

Carlson, E.A. 2004. *Mendel's Legacy: the Origin of Classical Genetics*. Cold Spring Harbor, NY.: Cold Spring Harbor Laboratory.

Chan, H.F.; Frey, B.S.; Gallus, J. et al. 2014. 'Academic honors and performance'. *Labour Economics* 31: 188–204.

Chityil, G. 2012. *Nobel Quotes: Inspiring and Perplexing Quotes of Nobel Prize Winners*. CreateSpace Independent Publishing Platform.

Christensen, M.L. 1997. *Heroes and Saints: More Stories about People who Made a Difference*. Louisville, KY: Westminster John Knox Press.

Coventry, P.A. and Pickstone, J.V. 1999. 'From what and why did genetics emerge as a medical specialism in the 1970s in the UK?'. *Social Science & Medicine* 49: 1227–1238.

Crawford, E.T. 1984. *The Beginnings of the Nobel Institution: the Science Prizes, 1901–1915*. Cambridge and Paris: Cambridge University Press and Editions de la Maison de l'Homme.

Crawford, E.T. 2002a. *The Nobel Population; A Census of the Nominators and Nominees for the Prizes in Physics and Chemistry, 1901–1950*. Tokyo: Universal Academy Press.

Crawford, E.T. 2002b. *Historical Studies in the Nobel* Archives. Tokyo: Universal Academy Press.

Dingle, C.A. 2012. *Memorable Quotations: Nobel Prize Winners of the Past.* Kindle E-book.

Ferry, G. and Sulston, J. 2002. *The Common Thread: A Story of Science, Politics, Ethics and the Human Genome.* Washington, DC: Joseph Henry Press.

Fleck, L. 1979. *The Genesis and Development of a Scientific Fact.* Chicago: University of Chicago Press.

Frey, B.S. and Gallus, J. 2015. 'Awards, honours, and ribbons: Between fame and shame'. *Vox,* March 11. https://www.bsfrey.ch/articles/D_261_2015.pdf (accessed January 10, 2019).

Frey, B.S. and Gallus, J. 2017. *Honours versus Money: the Economics of Awards.* Oxford: Oxford University Press.

Goode, W.J. 1978. *The Celebration of Heroes: Prestige as a Control System.* Berkeley; Los Angeles; London: University of California Press.

Grmek, M.D. 1981. 'A plea for freeing the history of scientific discoveries from myth'. In *On Scientific Discovery: The Erice Lectures 1977. Boston Studies in the Philosophy and History of Science no. 34,* edited by M.D. Grmek, R.S. Cohen, G. Cimino, 9–42. Dordrecht and Boston: Reidel.

Grmek, M.D. 1999. 'La troisième revolution scientifique'. *Revue médicale de la Suisse romande* 119: 955–959.

Grmek, M.D. 2001. 'Revolutions dans l'histoire de la pensée biomédicale'. In *La vie, les maladies, et l'histoire,* edited by M.D. Grmek and L.L. Lambrichs, 47–49. Paris: Seuil.

Haddad, G.E. 1999. 'Medicine and the culture of commemoration: representing Robert Koch's discovery of the tubercle bacillus'. *Osiris* 14: 118–137.

Howell, J.D. 1995. *Technology in the Hospital: Transforming Patient Care in the Early Twentieth Century.* Baltimore: Johns Hopkins University Press.

Hua, M.J. 2016. *'Magic Bullets from Chinese Herbs. Transcription and the Making of Qinghao History,'* Master's Thesis, Anthropology, University of Chicago.

Improbable Research. 'About the Ig* Nobel Prizes', http://www.improbable.com/ig (accessed January 10, 2019).

Judson, H. 1979. *The Eighth Day of Creation: Makers of the Revolution in Biology.* New York: Simon and Schuster.

Judson, H. 2004. *The Great Betrayal: Fraud in Science.* Orlando: Harcourt.

Kantha, S.S. 1995. 'Is Karl Landsteiner the Einstein of the biomedical sciences?'. *Medical Hypotheses* 44: 254–256.

Keller, E.F. 2000. *The Century of the Gene.* Cambridge, Mass.: Harvard University Press.

Kevles, B. 1999. *Naked to the Bone: Medical Imaging in the Twentieth Century.* New Brunswick, N.J.: Rutgers University Press.

Kevles, D.J. 1985. *In the Name of Eugenics: Genetics and the Uses of Human Heredity.* New York: Knopf.

Kevles, D.J. and Hood, L. 1992. *The Code of Codes; Scientific and Social Issues in the Human Genome Project*. Cambridge, Mass.: Harvard University Press.

Kevles, D.J. 1998. *The Baltimore Case: a Trial of Politics, Science, and Character*. New York and London: Norton.

Kingston, W. 2004. 'Streptomycin, Schatz v. Waksman, and the balance of credit for discovery'. *Journal of the History of Medicine & Allied Sciences* 59: 441–462.

Kuhn, T.S. 1962. *The Structure of Scientific Revolutions*. Chicago: University of Chicago Press.

Lind, J. 1753. *Treatise on the Scurvy*. Edinburgh: Sands, Murray and Cochran.

Lindahl, B.I. 1992. 'Discovery, theory change, and the Nobel Prize: on the mechanisms of scientific evolution. An introduction'. *Theoretical Medicine* 13: 97–116.

Luttenberger, F. 1996. 'Excellence and chance: the Nobel Prize; case of E. Von Behring and É. Roux'. *History and Philosophy of the Life Sciences* 18: 225–239.

Mayr, E. 1982. *The Growth of Biological Thought; Diversity, Evolution, Inheritance*. Cambridge, Mass.: Belknap Press.

McCarthy, M. 1997. 'Nobel Prize winner Gajdusek admits child abuse'. *Lancet* 349: 623.

McLaren, A. 1990. *Our Own Master Race: Eugenics in Canada, 1885–1945*. Toronto: McClelland and Stewart.

Merton, R.K. 1973. *The Sociology of Science: Theoretical and Empirical Investigations*. Chicago and London: University of Chicago Press.

Nye, M.J. 2006. 'Scientific biography: history of science by another means'. *Isis* 97 (2): 322–329.

Ogburn, W.F. and Thomas, D. 1922. 'Are inventions inevitable?'. *Political Science Quarterly* 37: 83–98.

Olby, R.C. 1974. *The Path to the Double Helix*. Seattle: University of Washington.

Plotz, D. 2005. *The Genius Factory: the Curious History of the Nobel Prize Sperm Bank*. New York: Random House.

Prasad, A. 2007. 'The amorphous anatomy of an invention: the case of magnetic resonance imaging (MRI)'. *Social Studies of Science* 37: 533–560.

Pratt, D. 2016. 'From suffering, adversity to the Nobel Prize'. *San Diego Jewish World*, 29 July. http://www.sdjewishworld.com/2016/07/29/from-suffering-adversity-to-the-nobel-prize (accessed January 10, 2019).

Proctor, R. 1988. *Racial Hygiene: Medicine under the Nazis*. Cambridge, Mass: Harvard University Press.

Redelmeier, R.J. and Naylor C.D. 2016. 'Changes in characteristics and time to recognition of medical scientists awarded a Nobel Prize'. *JAMA* 316 (19): 2043–2044.

Risse, G.B. 1999. *Mending Bodies, Saving Souls: a History of Hospitals*. New York: Oxford.

Rogers, K. 2011. *Medicine and Healers through History*. New York: Britannica Educational Publishing.

Sapp, J. 1990. 'The nine lives of Gregor Mendel'. In *Experimental Inquiries: Historical, Philosophical and Social Studies of Experimentation in Science*, edited by H.E. LeGrand, 137–166. Dordrecht: Kluwer Academic Publishers.

Sinclair, L. 2008. 'Recognizing, understanding and treating pernicious anemia'. *Journal of the Royal Society of Medicine* 101 (5): 262–264.

Stevens, R. 1999. *In Sickness and in Wealth: American Hospitals in the Twentieth Century*. Baltimore: Johns Hopkins University Press.

Söderqvist, T. 2007. *The History and Poetics of Scientific Biography*. Aldershot: Ashgate.

Wainwright, M. 1991. 'Streptomycin: discovery and resultant controversy'. *History and Philosophy of the Life Sciences* 13: 97–124.

Weksler, M.E. 2004. 'Naming Streets for Physicians: "l'affaire Carrel"'. *Perspectives in Biology & Medicine* 47: 67–73.

Wuchty, S.; Jones, B.F.; Uzzi, B. 2007. 'The increasing dominance of teams in the production of knowledge'. *Science* 316: 1036–1039.

Yarborough, M. and Sharp, R.R. 2009. 'Public trust and research a decade later: What have we learned since Jesse Gelsinger's death?'. *Molecular Genetics and Metabolism* 97 (1): 4–5.

YourNobelPrize, http://krboerup.wixsite.com/yournobelprize (accessed January 10, 2019)

Zuckerman, H. 1967. 'Nobel laureates in science: patterns of productivity, collaboration, and authorship'. *American Sociological Review* 32: 391–403.

Zuckerman, H. 1978. 'The sociology of the Nobel Prize: further notes and queries'. *American Scientist* 66: 420–425.

Zuckerman, H. 1992. 'The proliferation of prizes: Nobel complements and Nobel surrogates in the reward system of science'. *Theoretical Medicine* 13: 217–231.

Zuckerman, H. 1996. *Scientific Elite: Nobel Laureates in the United States*. New Brunswick, N.J.: Transaction Publishers.

Zwart, H. 2008. 'Understanding the Human Genome Project: a biographical approach'. *New Genetics and Society* 27 (4): 353–376.

CHAPTER 2

More Than a Prize: The Creation of the Nobel System

Gustav Källstrand

In this chapter, I argue for the importance of viewing the institutions responsible for the Nobel Prize as a 'Nobel system' – understood as a process of inter-related institutions, organizations and individuals – in which the parts are entangled in several ways, not least financially. By looking at how the Nobel Foundation and the prize awarding institutions dealt with constructing and financing buildings and research institutions, I make the case that the Nobel System was from the outset a construction where the parts tried to gain autonomy, and that they did this by using the Nobel funds as a resource. This acquired legitimacy by referring to an ideological 'ultimate end' of the Nobel Prize that transcended the awarding of a prize.

More Than a Prize

According to the *Encyclopedia Britannica,* the Nobel Prize is 'widely regarded as the most prestigious award given for intellectual achievement in the world'.[1] This is a status that the Nobel Foundation does not take for granted, but is constantly working on. They work to ensure financial support for the prize awarding institution's thorough investigation process of potential laureates. Since the 1990s, the Foundation has also embarked on a program of outreach activities through the establishing of a museum and a media company. These activities can be seen as 'legitimizing devices' for the prize.[2]

This is in keeping with what brand management researchers Mats Urde and Stephen Greyser call 'stewardship' in the management of a 'corporate heritage brand' like the Nobel Prize.[3] They say that the Nobel Prize is not only a brand with a history, but also that the history is a crucial part of its identity. This plays out in the attitude within the Nobel system that the prize has received its

---

1 https://www.britannica.com/topic/Nobel-Prize (accessed February 26, 2019).
2 Lovell 2006, 44.
3 Urde and Greyser 2015, 319.

status through its track record, and that the preservation of this tradition is the most important task of the system.[4]

However, the prize does not only represent a list of previous laureates. It also represents values having to do with the phrase in Alfred Nobel's will about awarding those who have 'conferred the greatest benefit to mankind', and it becomes symbol of a set of cultural values that is not always clearly defined but which centers around the possibilities of science, culture and politics to affect society in a positive way.[5] This work is accelerating presently with the expansion of Nobel Media and the construction of a Nobel Center. There is a view that the Nobel Prize carries meaning that transcends the awarding of prizes. In the Foundation's Annual Review it is described as being 'entrusted with managing and carefully developing the trademarks and intangible assets that have been built up during the more than century-long history of the Nobel Prize'.[6] Today, this means to 'maintain its position and further develop its activities'.[7] But the view that the Nobel Foundation should have 'activities' beyond giving away prizes means that the Nobel Prize is an institution actively building its own reputation and renown.

The view that the prize has a goal beyond 'just' giving a prize to deserving persons is not new. In the statutes of the Foundation from 1900 there was a section that says Nobel's funds can be used to 'promote the purposes the donor ultimately intended' by other means than awarding prizes.[8] What I want to look at in this paper is what this meant when it was written – and furthermore how this was used when the Nobel system went through its first three formative decades. For this, it is necessary to look at the Nobel Prize as the result of relationships within an organizational structure that is far from monolithic.

The Creation of the Nobel System

Urde and Greyser refer to the prize as 'processes of interrelated institutions, organizations and individuals'.[9] I refer to this process as the 'Nobel system', a phrase often used by people working with the prize as a useful (and time-saving)

---

4   Urde and Greyser 2015, 324.
5   Urde and Greyser 2015, 325–326.
6   The Nobel Foundation Annual Report 2015 (The Nobel Foundation, 2016), 4.
7   The Nobel Foundation Annual Review 2013 (The Nobel Foundation, 2014), 7.
8   'Grundstadgar för Nobelstiftelsen; gifna Stockholms slott den 29 juni 1900' in *Svensk för-fattning-samling Nr. 63 1900* (1900), 3. Transl. by author, in original: 'till att annorledes än genom prisutdelning främja de ändamål testator ytterst afsett'.
9   Urde and Greyser 2015, 322.

way of describing a complex and sometimes nebulous organizational structure. The Nobel system consists of two major parts: the Nobel Foundation and the prize awarding institutions (the Royal Academy of Sciences, the Karolinska Institute, the Swedish Academy and the Norwegian Nobel Committee, selected by the Norwegian parliament Stortinget). The role of the Nobel Foundation is to manage the financial means left by Alfred Nobel, which means to secure the financial means for the prize money and for the work of the prize awarding institutions in selecting the recipients.[10]

There is an inherent tension in this system. The prize awarding institutions feel a strong sense of propriety over the prize, while the Nobel Foundation is legally and financially responsible for it. This creates a situation where it has not always been clear who has an overreaching responsibility for the prize. For the Nobel system itself, this can be complicated enough, but for outsiders it creates a situation where commentary and criticism can be misguided because of a lack of understanding of this complex system.[11] So how was this system created?

After Alfred Nobel's death negotiations started with the prize awarding institutions, in order to set up the rules for the prize and the management of Nobel's fortune. The prize awarders were – with the exception of Stortinget – hesitant.[12] The explicit reason was that they could not accept this task until they were sure that an organization was in place for selecting laureates. Less explicit was the fact that they saw Nobel's donation as a possibility to benefit their own institutions, and that they would not agree until they made sure that they benefited from it. Chief among these benefits was the establishment of the Nobel Institutes. These were institutions where experts would help the prize awarding institutions in their evaluation of candidates for the prize.[13] For the scientific institutions these were a way to ensure access to scientific facilities and revenue to keep these going.[14] For the Swedish Academy, the institute was a way to elevate their status to a more scientific level, and for the Norwegian Nobel Committee the institute fulfilled the basic need of creating an organizational basis for the committee.[15]

---

10   'Grundstadgar för Nobelstiftelsen; gifna Stockholms slott den 29 juni 1900' in *Svensk för-fattning-samling Nr. 63 1900* (1900), 6.
11   Lindqvist 2011.
12   Sohlman 2001; Falnes 1938, 135–136.
13   Crawford 1984, 66, 69–70, 73–75; Rydén 2011, 188, 544–545, 723; Protokoll hållna vid sammanträden för öfverläggning om Alfred Nobels testamente (Stockholm: P.A. Norstedts och söner 1899), 7–9, 116–118.
14   Friedman 1990.
15   Libæk 2000, 8–9; Rydén 2011, 188, 544–545, 723.

The Swedish press picked up on the Nobel Institutes, and their reactions speak to how widespread the view was that the prize was more than 'just' a prize. The papers wrote that although the prize was anticipated, the real pay-off from the Nobel donation was the institutes' potential to make Stockholm a center for international science.[16] Since both the prize awarders and the public opinion were in favor of these institutes, there was no discussion raised on whether it was acceptable to use the donation of Alfred Nobel for research institutes which were not mentioned in his will. Instead this was just seen as one among many alterations made to the will when it was transformed from its original state to the statutes of a complex institution.

The Nobel Palace

When the Nobel Foundation was created, a sum of 1,5 million kronor (the equivalent of roughly $340,000 in 1901 and $10 million today) was set aside for the construction of the Nobel Institutes. At the same time, a special fund was created to finance a building for the Foundation itself, of 900,000 kronor, a fund that would grow since royalties from some of Nobel's patents was tied to it. This building was meant to house the Foundation's administration (some ten people) and a large lecture hall where the award ceremony could be held. Hope was that the Institutes and the Foundation's building would be placed together, thus creating the physical representation of a unified Nobel System.[17]

The Foundation waited to gauge the reactions to this among the prize awarding institutions, but when it soon became clear that they would rather use the Nobel funds to strengthen their own organizations it started planning for its own building.[18] After a few years of negotiations the Foundation was able to secure a tract of land close at the end of the newly constructed Strand-vägen.[19] This was a fashionable street running along the water from the city center to the bridge to Djurgården, an island that was partly a royal park but also home to the Nordiska Museum and Skansen, two important institutions

---

16   Källstrand 2012, 45, 288.
17   'Grundstadgar för Nobelstiftelsen; gifna Stockholms slott den 29 juni 1900' in *Svensk för-fattning-samling Nr. 63 1900* (1900), 5, 9; Draft of letter to the Nobel Board of Trustees June 7 1901, supplement to the Nobel Foundation Board Meetings 1900–1901; Nobel Foundation Board Meetings 1902, 12–13.
18   Nobel Foundation Board Meetings 1906, 11.
19   Källstrand 2012, 177–179; Sörenson 1992, 173–174, 194, 208; Nobel Foundation Board Meet-ings 1905, 44–45, 57–59, 64–66, Nobel Foundation Board Meetings 1906, 23, 47–48, 72–73; Nobel Foundation Board Meetings 1908, 13–14.

for the creation of a national Swedish identity at the turn of the century. In this setting, the Nobel building would be perceived as an important public building and even though it would not physically be a center for the different Nobel Institutes it would be a symbol of unity for the Nobel institution as a whole.[20]

The Foundation commissioned Ferdinand Boberg, one of Sweden's most famous architects at the time, to draw a building with a lecture hall that would seat between 1600 and 2000 persons.[21] The design was presented to the public in 1911, and a long discussion ensued. While there were many critics of Boberg's style, few critics questioned the purpose of the building. Indeed, the 'Nobel Palace' was welcomed as the next logical step in the development of the Nobel institution.[22] In the end, however, the plans were rejected. This had less to do with the criticism than with the size and the cost of the palace.[23]

What did the Nobel Foundation wish to express with this Nobel palace? It was a very large building, dominated on the outside by a central tower and on the inside by a large hall for the celebrations, which could be also be used for concerts. Its main entrance was to be used only by the Royal family, the Nobel laureates and representatives from the Nobel system – other guests were to enter through the backdoors. And although it was large, the palace did not have space for the administration of the Foundation, which was placed in a smaller adjacent building. That the festivities were more important than the scientific content became clear by the fact that the ceremonial hall was thought to be too large for the Nobel lectures, which were to be held in the public entrance foyer. The interior was to be painted in dark colors, with occasional gold details. It was to be decorated with classical symbols, previous Nobel laureates and the Swedish royal family – a way to frame the prize as something deeply rooted in a historical tradition.[24]

What this building conveyed to the public was that the Nobel Prize was something very solemn and high-brow. It did not refer to the prizes connection to modern science or literature, but rather to a long tradition of classical *Bildung*. This message did not originate with Boberg, who just followed the lead given by the award ceremonies that had been held in the Musical Academy in Stockholm since 1901, and which also drew on nationalism and tradition for legitimacy.[25] The Nobel Palace was an expression of the Nobel Foundation's

---

20   Källstrand 2012, 164–165.
21   *Handlingar rörande Nobelstiftelsens byggnadsfråga* (Nobel Foundation, 1912), 5–21, 25–42.
22   Källstrand 2012, 126–127.
23   Sörensson 1992, 204–205; Nobel Foundation Board Meetings 1912, 12.
24   *Handlingar rörande Nobelstiftelsens byggnadsfråga* (Nobelstiftelsen, 1912), 9, 27–28, 36–37, 40–41.
25   Källstrand 2012, 126–127.

ambition to make the Nobel Prize part of the Swedish public life, and to make an impression on foreign dignitaries and press when they came to Stockholm for the Nobel festivities. What we see is the will to make the prize into a symbol of something more than just the work of each years' individual Nobel laureates.

The First Nobel Institutes

The first two Nobel Institutes were not scientific ones. Instead, they belonged to the Swedish Academy and the Norwegian Nobel Committee. There is some irony here, in that the Institutes originated with the idea that committees should have laboratories in which to test the candidates' work. However, the need for assistance in evaluating candidates was felt perhaps to a larger extent in these two institutions. The Swedish Academy was a literary academy devoted to the Swedish language. It needed to expand its competence in the field of modern international literature in order to carry out its task.[26] In Norway the Nobel Committee decided – after a few years of discussion – to build a Nobel Institute which was to serve as a library and as a research institution for the experts that the committee enlisted to help them with evaluations.[27] The Swedish Academy's institute was a composite of two parts, one devoted to literary studies and the other a library. They were housed together and opened in January 1901. The Norwegian Institute was founded in 1904 and received its own building in 1905.

The Royal Academy of Sciences started planning for two Nobel Institutes, one in physics and one in chemistry. The Academy was at this time involved in a project creating a 'science city' on the northern outskirts of Stockholm. Both a new building for the Academy and a new Museum of Natural History would be placed here, amongst other research institutes. Two Nobel Institutes would be a perfect fit.[28] However, things took an unexpected turn when the physical chemist Svante Arrhenius, a member of the Academy and a professor at the Stockholm Högskola announced that he had been offered a position in Berlin which he was inclined to accept unless a better position could be offered in Sweden. The Academy, keen to keep Arrhenius who was a prestigious researcher, a key factor in the Nobel Committees for physics and chemistry, and himself a Nobel laureate in chemistry, decided to create the Nobel Institute for

---

26   Rydén 2011, 188, 544–545, 723; Nobel Foundation Board Meetings 1900–1901, 42.
27   Libaeck 2000.
28   Beckman 1999, 128–136; Eriksson 1989, 91.

Physical Chemistry for Arrhenius.[29] The message was clear: the prize awarding institutions saw the Nobel funds as a solution to their own immediate needs rather than as the basis of a new institution.

This also meant that the Nobel Institute became a small laboratory. At first housed in an apartment in the same house in which he lived, it later became a one-man institution where the director was the center both as a professional and as a private person. It also combined living quarters with a work space. This set up was part of a European tradition, where individuals networked by visiting each other's home-laboratories.[30] Although this was in contradiction with the ambition of making the Nobel Institutes large-scale scientific environments, it was something that the Academy both needed and could afford. The 300,000 kronor allotted for the institutes might be sufficient to erect a building, but not to finance its running expenses. This conclusion was also reached at the Karolinska Institute, where the members decided to wait for a better financial situation.[31]

The Great War Changes the Landscape

During the fall of 1914 there was a discussion within the prize awarding institutions that spilled over into the public sphere: should the Nobel Prize be awarded during wartime? Those in favor of awarding the prize saw it as a symbol for the international spirit in science and literature, whereas those opposed argued that the prize to any given country might be seen as a support for that nation (see also Sven Widmalm's chapter in this volume). Both views hinged on neutrality, and as Sven Widmalm has shown, science and neutrality were closely linked concepts at this time in Sweden.[32]

There were no grounds in the statutes for reserving the prize on account of the war, but the Foundation and the prize awarders decided to ask the government for an exception to the rules, allowing them to postpone the decision until the next year. This was something else than reserving the prize – to do that still required a decision that none of the candidates could be considered worthy. The decision was postponed until 1915, a technical solution that meant that no candidates were evaluated or rejected in 1914.[33] This was done in the

---

29   Crawford 1996, 217.
30   Bergwik 2014, 267, 276.
31   Luttenberger, 1997, 3.
32   Widmalm 2012, 66; *Aftonbladet* September 6, 7, 11 1914; *Svenska Dagbladet* September 7, November 5, October 31, December 7 1914.
33   Nobel Foundation Board Meetings 1914, 46, 50–51.

hope that the war would be over quickly, but since this was not the case, the matter was just delayed one year.[34] Just as public opinion was divided, so too were the prize awarding institutions. They did not agree on a coherent strategy for awarding prizes during the war. Indeed, they changed their own view from year to year, leaving the prize records for these year a patchwork of reserved, postponed and awarded prizes (Table 2.1.).

TABLE 2.1 Reserved and cancelled Nobel Prizes 1914–1938. In years not in the table, all prizes were awarded as usual. An important note is that the money from a reserved prize was placed in the prize awarders' special funds, meaning that they could get the interest from the sum.

	Physics	Chemistry	Physiology of medicine
1914	1914 reserved	1914 reserved	1914 reserved
1915	1914 and 1915 awarded	1914 and 1915 awarded	1914 awarded, 1915 reserved
1916	1916 reserved	1916 reserved	1915 cancelled, 1916 reserved
1917	1916 cancelled, 1917 reserved	1916 cancelled, 1917 reserved	1916 cancelled, 1917 reserved
1918	1917 awarded, 1918 reserved	1917 awarded, 1918 reserved	1917 cancelled, 1918 reserved
1919	1918 and 1919 awarded	1918 awarded, 1919 reserved	1918 cancelled, 1919 reserved
1920	1920 awarded	1919 cancelled, 1920 reserved	1919 and 1920 awarded
1921	1921 reserved	1920 awarded, 1921 cancelled	1921 reserved
1922	1921 awarded, 1922 awarded	1921 awarded, 1922 awarded	1921 cancelled, 1922 reserved
1924	1924 reserved	1924 reserved	1924 awarded
1925	1924 awarded, 1925 reserved	1924 cancelled, 1925 reserved	1925 reserved
1926	1925 and 1926 awarded	1925 and 1926 awarded	1925 cancelled, 1926 reserved
1927	1927 awarded	1927 reserved	1926 and 1927 awarded

---

34 Friedman 2001, 87–88; *Stockholms Dagblad* October 13, 21 1915; *Stockholms Tidningen* October 18 1915.

	Physics	Chemistry	Physiology of medicine
1928	1928 reserved	1927 and 1928 awarded	1928 awarded
1929	1928 and 1929 awarded	1929 awarded	1929 awarded
1931	1931 reserved	1931 awarded	1931 awarded
1932	1931 cancelled, 1932 reserved	1932 awarded	1932 awarded
1933	1932 and 1933 awarded	1933 reserved	1933 awarded
1934	1934 reserved	1933 cancelled, 1934 awarded	1934 awarded
1935	1934 cancelled, 1935 awarded	1935 awarded	1935 awarded
1938	1938 awarded	1938 cancelled (awarded in 1939)	1938 cancelled (awarded in 1939)

Cancelling the prizes had a very tangible financial consequence. The money for a prize that was not awarded could, according to the statutes, be placed in the special fund that the Foundation had set aside for each prize awarding institution. According to science historian Robert Marc Friedman this was an important part of the rationale for the decision to cancel so many prizes during the war.[35] Regardless of the motives, at the end of the war the prize awarders found themselves with a financial resource that they had not had a few years earlier.

At the Karolinska Institute, this awakened a new hope for a Nobel Institute. The proposal for an institute in physiology already came in late 1917. The idea was to create a smaller institution that could later be expanded. A counter-proposal for an institute for racial biology was made shortly thereafter. This was discussed but not pursued, partly because racial biology was not included in Nobel's will, but also because racial biology was deemed to be of national importance and therefore deserving of a larger government-funded institute (which it indeed got a few years later).[36] The proposal was then discussed and elaborated from 1919 to 1922. The idea was now that there would be two departments, one for physiology and one for pathology. While this did create some criticism on the grounds that this would limit the scope of the institutions, the main question was whether a Nobel Institute on the planned scale was

---

35   Friedman 2001, 94–95.
36   Luttenberger 1997, 5; Ambosiani 2009.

financially feasible.[37] There had been plans at the Royal Academy of Sciences for a department for cosmic physics at the Nobel Institute, but these were postponed already in 1918 for lack of funding (and not revived later).[38]

Immediately after the war, several Swedish scientists and intellectuals (amongst them Svante Arrhenius and the prime minister Hjalmar Branting) thought that the Nobel Prize might play an important role in rebuilding the severed ties in the international scientific community.[39] These ideas were present at Karolinska Institute, although the matter cannot be reduced to a question of an internationalist ethos: it was also a matter of using the Nobel Prize as a – in the words of historian of science Franz Luttenberger – 'scientific resource'.[40]

Finding More Ways to Use the Nobel Funds as a Financial Resource

The money from the cancelled Nobel Prizes were not the only resource available after the war. When Ferdinand Boberg's design was deemed too expensive, the question of a building for the Nobel Foundation lay dormant until late 1918, when it was decided that the Foundation should not build on such a monumental scale. A new City Hall and a Concert Hall were under way in Stockholm, and either of these ought to be suitable for the award ceremony. Free from the need to build a lecture hall, the Foundation quickly purchased a smaller office building for its administration – which meant that only about half of the resources allocated to the building funds would be needed.[41] The remainder was meant to be reinserted into the main fund of the Nobel Foundation.[42] This was welcome, since the fund had diminished due to both high inflation during the war and higher taxes. This led to the steady decrease of the Nobel Prize funds, a problem that both the Foundation and the prize awarding institutions wanted to remedy.[43] Ivar Afzelius, professor of law and member of the Swedish Academy, put forth the idea that the prize awarding institutions should all agree to raise the prize by abstaining from choosing a laureate one year, and return the prize money into the main fund.[44] This idea was soon turned into ways to increase funding for the Nobel Institutes. The basis

37   Luttenberger 1997, 4, 6–7.
38   Friedman 2001, 147.
39   Widmalm 1995, 345, 354–355, 359.
40   Luttenberger 1997, *passim*.
41   Nobel Foundation Board Meetings 1918, 63–65, 77–80.
42   Nobel Foundation Board Meetings 1920, 96–97.
43   Nobel Foundation Board Meetings 1927, 38–39.
44   Nobel Foundation Board Meetings 1920, 32–33, 44–45.

for these plans came from Svante Arrhenius. He first proposed that the money from the building project ought not to be moved to the main fund, but rather to the Nobel Institutes. And he went further. To ensure a continuing revenue, Arrhenius also argued that the money for the institute should be transferred from the Foundation to the Royal Academy of Science, which, contrary to the Foundation, was exempt from taxes.[45]

The discussion in the Foundation resulted in two proposals in 1921. The first was that out of the 2,5 million kronor in the fund, 1,5 should be divided and transferred to the prize awarding institutions. Since this was not supported in the statutes, permission from government was needed and indeed applied for. The chancellor of justice, however, raised objections against using Nobel's funds to finance the prize awarding institutions beyond the recompense it received for selecting the laureates, and the proposition was denied.[46] A second proposal was that 1 million should go to the main fund and only 500,000 kronor to the prize awarders.[47] When this was put to the prize awarding institutions, however, only the Swedish Academy and the Norwegian Nobel Committee accepted. This is hardly surprising, since it represented a setback for the Karolinska and the Royal Swedish Academy of Sciences, and they probably wanted to keep their options open for another solution in the future.

The key player during these discussions at the Karolinska Institute was the chairman of the Nobel Committee for Physiology of Medicine, J.E. Johansson. He was a strong supporter of the Nobel Institute, as well as a close friend (and indeed brother in law) to Svante Arrhenius. Johansson first argued that the building fund should be used for the Nobel Institutes rather than be placed in the main fund. According to him, the decreasing prize amount was not a problem since the prestige of the prize depended on the integrity of the evaluation process rather than the money. All available funds should therefore be placed at the hands of the prize awarders, for them to use as they saw fit to strengthen the evaluation process.[48]

In early 1923, the director of the Nobel Foundation, Henrik Sederholm, wrote a critical memorandum, analyzing Johansson's proposal. Sederholm stated that it was obvious that the purpose of such a fund would be to support the Nobel Institutes, and this was not in keeping with Alfred Nobel's will. This is quite interesting, since it goes against the general agreement that Nobel had had an ultimate purpose with his prize that could be reached by other means

---

45   Svante Arrhenius to the Royal Academy of Sciences 14th April and 16th October 1920, supplements to Nobel Foundation Board Meetings 1920.

46   Nobel Foundation Board Meetings 1921, 61–62.

47   Nobel Foundation Board Meetings 1922, 19–20.

48   Luttenberger 1997, 8–9; Nobel Foundation Board Meetings 1921, 30–31.

than the prize. Sederholm quite frankly stated that the purpose of Nobel's will was to award prizes – not to support the prize awarding institutions. However, this was not an ideological shift but a reference to the views that the chancellor of justice had brought up in 1921.[49] The Foundation's board agreed with Sederholm's statement, and no further mention of this idea can be found in the minutes of the board meetings.[50]

This was a setback for Johansson. He still supported the idea of a Nobel Institute, however, and suggested that it might be possible to create a preliminary and more modest institute with only one or two employees, that could function for a few years while the funds grew.[51] This was similar to the arrangements made by the Royal Academy of Sciences for the Nobel Institute for Physical Chemistry.[52] But the difference was that while Arrhenius was content with his one man-institute, Johansson wanted the Nobel Institutes to become a research environment where experts from several various disciplines worked.[53] Johansson returned to Afzelius' original proposal on how to increase the Nobel funds: cancelling prizes. A better way, he said, to use these funds could scarcely be imagined than to 'maintain scientific institutions devoted to securing the future prize selection'.[54] According to his calculations four out of ten prizes should be withheld to secure the necessary funds.[55] Looking at the prize records for the years when he was the chairman of the Nobel Committee, we can see that he may well have put this logic in action. Between 1919 and 1926, two out of eight prizes were withheld, and this number might have been higher, since the prize for 1926 was awarded retrospectively in 1927, after Johansson had resigned as chairman.[56]

Of course the case can be made that this was because Johansson wanted the committee to raise the scientific standards for the prize, and thus found it harder to find worthy candidates. However, this becomes less credible in light

49   Memorandum from Henrik Sederholm 20th March 1923, supplement to the Nobel Foundation Board Meetings 1923.

50   Luttenberger, 1997, 9; Liljestrand 1960, 574, 576; Nobel Foundation Board Meetings 1923, 30. In a history of the Karolinska, a chairman of the Nobel Committee, Göran Liljestrand, claims that 300,000 SEK was paid to each institution in 1922. No evidence of this can be found in the archives, and the date seems odd since the question was apparently still debated in the Foundation in early 1923.

51   Johansson 1926, 80–82; Luttenberger 1997, 9.

52   Källstrand 2012, 171.

53   Johansson 1926, 80–81.

54   Johansson 1926, 82.

55   Luttenberger 1997, 10.

56   Luttenberger 1997, 11.

of the many statements Johansson made to the effect that prizes should be withheld for financial reasons.[57] This shows that although the question seems to have been dropped from the official agenda in 1922, the idea that the Nobel funds could be used for something more than only for the prize was still present at Karolinska for a long time.

Tax Exemption

In 1904, the liberal member of parliament Carl Lindhagen suggested in Swedish parliament that the Nobel Foundation should be exempt from taxes. Lindhagen knew the Nobel Foundation well since he, in his capacity as legal counsel to the executors of the will, had drafted its statutes. The background to his motion was that the prize sum had been decreasing since the inception of the Foundation due to its heavy tax burden. He argued that keeping the Nobel Prize at a high level would benefit Sweden more than the revenues taxing the Foundation. The opponents claimed that the prize did not have such a big influence on the international image of Sweden, that the Foundation was not a scientific academy and could thus not be exempt from taxes.[58]

Linhagen's motion did not pass. Until the war the taxes were still felt to be tolerable, but when inflation and a general decline in the economy coincided with raised taxes, the Foundation felt that they needed to act in this matter again. An investigation was carried out in 1920 by a legal expert, David Davidsson. He pointed out that although the Nobel Foundation might not be an 'academy or scientific society' in the traditional sense, it would be possible to argue that the Nobel Foundation was scientific in the sense that it was responsible for a scientific task: the awarding of prizes in science. The Nobel Foundation was unusual in that its scientific tasks were carried out not by its own members but by other scientific institutions.[59]

Davidsson's advice was that the Foundation should declare itself exempt from taxes on these grounds, and if the tax authorities did not accept this straight away, be prepared to argue the case in court.[60] This meant the start

---

57 *Dagens Nyheter* November 14 1925. See also *Nya Dagligt Allehanda* December 8th 1925, where S.E. Henschen claims that Johansson was explicit in his will to routinely reserve prizes, and that it was only after being informed that this was illegal that he dropped the suggestion.

58 Källstrand 2012, 99–101.

59 Memorandum from David Davidsson [undated, presented to the board January 29th, 1920], supplement to the Nobel Foundation Board Meetings 1920.

60 Nobel Foundation Board Meetings 1920, 17–19.

of a legal battle in which the Nobel Foundation claimed that it was a scientific institution and the tax authorities claimed that is was not.[61] This battle was highly visible in the press. Both the prize awarding institutions and the Nobel Foundation made sure that the public was aware that the Nobel Prize was diminishing in size because of taxes. They were successful in gaining support for their cause.[62] In 1924, the Nobel Foundation was actually granted a partial (but substantial) cut in their tax liability, from 1,5 million kronor to 300,000. However, in 1925 this decision was overturned by the Supreme Administrative Court.[63]

According to the law, the Nobel Foundation could not be seen as a scientific institution. However, this could still be changed by parliament through new legislation. In November Emanuel Nobel, one of Alfred Nobel's nephews, directly appealed to the government to make a change. He was seconded by the Nobel Foundation and the prize awarding institution.[64] Nobel claimed that the Nobel Foundation paid as much money in taxes as it awarded prizes. This message was picked up by the press, creating a very favorable atmosphere for the Nobel Foundation, although some complained that it was still problematic since it made Sweden look bad from an international perspective.[65] That year the prize awarding institutions did not award any prizes; a move generally thought to be in protest. A representative of the Karolinska was quite open about the fact that economic considerations had been part of the decision.[66]

The campaign proved successful. In January 1926, the Secretary of Finance stated that he would propose in parliament that taxes be lowered for the Foundation.[67] This motion became part of a broader discussion on the municipal taxes, but in early 1927 the Nobel Foundation was granted a partial tax exemption, enough to stabilize finances.[68] This decision would have important consequences for the Nobel Institutes.

---

61   Nobel Foundation Board Meetings 1921, 46–47, 82; 1922, 36, 52.
62   For instance *Dagens Nyheter* April 2nd 1922; *Svenska Dagbladet* October 27th 1923; *Dagens Nyheter* March 24 1925; *Svenska Dagbladet* May 3, September 25 1925.
63   Oddly, this was not reported in the Nobel Foundation Board Meetings, but it was reported in the press. See *Nya Dagligt Allehanda* January 2nd 1924; *Aftonbladet* January 2nd 1924; *Dagens Nyheter* April 22, 1925.
64   Nobel Foundation Board Meetings 1925, 69; see for instance *Svenska Dagbladet* November 12th 1925.
65   *Aftonbladet* October 2nd 1925; *Social-Demokraten* January 23rd 1926.
66   *Dagens Nyheter* November 14th, 15th 1925.
67   *Nya Dagligt Allehanda* January 12th 1926.
68   Nobel Foundation Board Meetings 1927, 37; *Stockholms Dagblad* February 26th 1927.

The Nobel Institutes in the 1930s

During the 1920s, the prize awarding institutions were able to use the special funds to finance research, often carried out by members of the prize awarding institutions and even the Nobel Committees.[69] In the 1930s, however, the Nobel Institutes finally became a reality. This was made possible by the developments we have seen in the Nobel Foundation, when in 1932 a proposal was made by the prize awarding institutions that the remaining 1,000,000 kronor in the building fund should be distributed among them.[70] This had not been possible in 1921, but now it could be done, for two reasons. The first was the partial tax exemption in 1927, and the second was that the question of a building for the Foundation had been solved. Although the Foundation had decided on a more modest building in 1918, this matter was not completely settled until 1926, since the building the Foundation had bought needed extensive renovation. In the end it was actually torn down and rebuilt, which meant that the Foundation could only start using it in 1926.[71] In that same year, the prize award ceremony was moved from the Musical Academy to the Concert Hall.[72] By 1932, the question of a building for the Foundation was thus resolved – and the funds could finally be put to the use of the prize awarding institutions.

The first new Nobel Institute was a modest one. Since the early 1920s, Carl Wilhelm Oseen, a member of the Nobel Committee for Physics had argued the need for an institute for theoretical physics. At that time, theoretical physics was seen as less prestigious than experimental physics, but that was about to change. Nobel Prizes to Max Planck, Albert Einstein and Niels Bohr paved the way. Then Svante Arrhenius passed away in 1927 and the Institute for Physical Chemistry ceased its activities. Together with Manne Siegbahn Oseen managed to convince the Royal Academy of Sciences to turn Arrhenius' institute into a Nobel Institute for Theoretical Physics, which opened its doors in 1933.[73] The same year, Paul Dirac, Erwin Schrödinger and Werner Heisenberg received their Nobel Prizes, a sign that theory was now accepted as an important part of physics.

At the same time, there was a shift in both physics and chemistry towards what Alvin Weinberg called 'Big Science' – an era ushered in by Ernst Lawrence's invention of the cyclotron in 1929. Many other researchers wanted to

---

69 Friedman 2001, 151–152.

70 Nobel Foundation Board Meetings 1932, 36–37, 45, 50, 60.

71 Nobel Foundation Board Meetings 1920, 40–41; 1923, 10–11, 16–17, 29, 34–35, 53–54; 1924, 1–2, 34, 42, 49, 52–53, 64, 68–71, 77, 83–84; 1925, 1–3, 53–55; 1926, 1–3, 60–61; 1927, 25, 1928, 19–20.

72 Nobel Foundation Board Meetings 1926, 77–79.

73 Friedman 2001, 215–217; Nobel Foundation Board Meetings 1933, 46–47.

emulate Lawrence's success, by creating scientific environment centered on this expensive piece of experimental equipment.[74] One of these was Manne Siegbahn, and to create an institute for isotope research he realized that he would need funding from several sources. While the Nobel fund might contribute to the construction of an institute, it would not be enough to pay for running expenses. For these Siegbahn managed to secure funding from the Knut and Alice Wallenberg fund, on condition that the Nobel money paid for the building, which succeeded in 1936.[75] This was all done under the auspices of the Royal Academy of Sciences, and the institute created was actually called the Royal Academy of Sciences Research Institute for Experimental Physics. Again, we see how a prize awarding institution used Nobel funding as a resource. And although the institute was not technically a Nobel Institute, Siegbahn and other researchers at the Institute could still receive grants from the special fund, among them the exiled Lise Meitner (famous for her theoretical work on nuclear fusion, and for not being awarded the Nobel Prize for this work in 1945 when the experimentalist Otto Hahn did receive it).[76]

What we also see is that the Nobel Foundation became part of the emerging landscape of funding bodies of Swedish science. This was the case at the Karolinska Institute, which finally received a Medical Nobel Institute in 1936. At this time, the Karolinska was going through an expansive phase, and the Nobel funds had already played a part in this through financial support from the special fund during the 1920s. One of the researchers who received substantial funding was Göran Liljestrand, often described as one of the chief architects behind the Karolinska transformation from a medical school to a research university.[77]

However, as in physics, the Nobel funds could not be the only source of revenue. Like most major research institutes, the Karolinska turned to the Rockefeller Foundation. In order to do this, it was important to show that the Karolinska was able to build a viable scientific environment, and the fact that there was a group of scientists working there, engaged in advanced research was helpful. The Nobel Institutes were also important here, as a sign of the general status of Swedish science. They were connected to successful individuals, which to the Rockefeller Foundation was a sign that the regular academic system in Sweden was unable to take care of talented researchers without

---

74   Hiltzik 2015, 45–47, 52–54, 121; Weinberg 1961.
75   Friedman 2001, 215–217; Nobel Foundation Board Meetings 1935, 53–54; 1936, 42–43, 71–72.
76   Nobel Foundation Board Meetings 1938, 67.
77   Ljungström 2010, 19–20, 26; Huldt, Normark & Norrving 2013, 70–73.

external support. At the same time, it showed that there was potential talent in need of means. From 1934, the Karolinska started to receive Rockefeller Funding, and this was an important step in the process towards becoming an internationally renowned research institution.[78]

Another key part was of course the creation of a dedicated research institute, and this was finally accomplished in 1936, when the decision for a Medical Nobel Institute was taken. The discussion had started the year before, when Liljestrand and Einar Hammarsten made the proposal for an institute for biochemistry, which was accepted by the Karolinska early in 1936. When this was presented to the Nobel Foundation, it sparked discussions that were largely practical and centered around how it was to be financed. The Foundation required the director of the institute to be involved in evaluating nominees for the Nobel Prize. This marks a clear difference between this institute and the one created for Manne Siegbahn – the Karolinska's was tied closer to the Nobel Foundation, or at least to the Nobel Prize. And while Siegbahn was employed by the Royal Academy of Sciences, the director of the Medical Nobel Institute, Hugo Theorell, was organizationally kept separate from the faculty at the Karolinska.[79]

In 1945, two more divisions of the Nobel Institute were created, one in neurophysiology and one in medical cell research and genetics. Both were financed only in part by Nobel funds, much like Siegbahn's institute. The Nobel means were enough to accomplish this without support from the Rockefeller Foundation, but their existence helped with the extensive investments that Rockefeller did instigate after World War II.[80] Regardless of the relative worth of the fund as a resource in itself or as 'seed money', the Nobel donation did play a role for the Nobel Prize awarding institution that transcended the importance of the prize.[81]

The Creation of the Nobel System

The view that the Nobel Prize has the potential to be more than 'just' a prize has deep roots in the system. We see this explicitly in the statutes of the Nobel Foundation, which stated that the money could be used to further the ultimate

---

78   Ljungström 2010, 82, 105, 122–125, 127.
79   Luttenberger 1997, 13; Ljungström 2010, 211–214; Nobel Foundation Board Meetings 1936, 48–50, 55–56, 92.
80   Ljungström 2010, 195.
81   Elzinga 1990, 236.

ends by other means than awarding prizes. What we saw during the 1920s was a period when the prize awarder really tested the limits of this rule. Would it be possible to decide not to award the prize in order to save money? As we have seen, there were a few pushbacks from the Swedish Chancellor of Justice, but these did not lead to any formal complaint. In spite of this, the prize awarders themselves cancelled this idea, but they did keep awarding large stipends for research. During the decade, the equivalent of roughly 10% of a Nobel Prize was given away by each prize awarder each year.

We have also seen that this may have played a role for the organization of science in Sweden, and particularly for the transformation of the Karolinska Institute into a research institution. For the prize awarders, it was quite clear that support for science was a worthy goal, and in line with the will of Alfred Nobel. This case was made simpler by the fact that the Nobel Institutes were created to assist the Nobel Committees in their evaluations. In this sense, the Nobel Institutes and the stipends from the special funds were not supporting the Karolinska Institute *per se*, but rather strengthening it as a part of the Nobel System.

The system was also important in a more practical sense, with capital being transferred between different funds inside the system to accommodate the needs that arose. The story of the Nobel Palace runs like a common thread through this whole history. In the beginning, it had been considered as a much needed unifying symbol for the whole Nobel System. However, the prize awarders would rather use the institutes to strengthen their own institution-building. When plans were put on hold during the war, the idea of a Nobel Palace became obsolete. The prize had become a symbol in its own right, and did not need the kind of physical representation of the Palace. This process took some time however. The attempts in the early 1920s by the prize awarding institutions to gain control of the funds reserved for the palace failed. A decade later, however, this was no longer a controversial issue. The money from this fund became the first contribution for new Nobel Institutes in the 1930s. The origin and enduring appeal of the Nobel Prize can only be fully understood by understanding its nature. It is not just a prize but a *system*, serving the general needs of Sweden and of global science, and the specific needs of Swedish research institutes.

Bibliography

Ambrosiani, A. 2009. *Professor Lennmalms förslag: Om 1918–1921 års diskussioner kring ett Nobelinstitut i rasbiologi vid Karolinska institutet.* Stockholm: Nobel Museum.

Beckman, J. 1999. *Naturens palats: Nybyggnad, vetenskap och utställning vid Naturhisto-riska riksmuseet 1866–1925*. Stockholm: Atlantis.

Bergwik, S. 2014. 'An assemblage of science and home: The gendered lifestyle of Svante Arrhenius and early-twentieth century physical chemistry'. *Isis* 105(2):264–291.

Crawford, E. 1984. *The Beginnings of the Nobel Institution: The Science Prizes 1901–1915*. Cambridge: Cambridge University Press.

Crawford, E. 1996. *Arrhenius: From Ionic Theory to Greenhouse Effect*. Canton, Mass.: Science History Publications.

Elzinga, A. 1990. 'Commentary'. In *Solomon's House Revisited: The Organization and In-stitutionalization of Science*, edited by Tore Frängsmyr. Canton, Mass.: Science History Publications.

Eriksson, G. 1989. 'The Academy in the daily life of Sweden'. In *Science in Sweden: The Royal Swedish Academy of Sciences 1739–1989*, edited by Tore Frängsmyr. Canton, Mass.: Science History Publications.

Falnes, O.J. 1938. *Norway and the Nobel Peace Prize*. New York: Columbia University Press.

Friedman, R.M. 1990. 'The Nobel Prizes and the Invigoration of Swedish Science'. In *Solomon's House Revisited: The Organization and Institutionalization of Science*, edited by Tore Frängsmyr. Canton, Mass.: Science History Publications.

Hiltzik, M. 2015. *Big Science: Ernest Lawrence and the Invention that Launched the Mili-tary-Industrial Complex*. New York: Simon & Shuster.

Huldt, I.; Normark, D.; Norrving, B. 2013. *Från läkarskola till medicinskt universitet: Karolinska institutets ledning 1953–2012*. Stockholm: Karolinska Institutet University Press.

Johansson, J.E. 1926. *Minneslista för Nobelprisgruppen i fysiologi eller medicin*. Stock-holm: Norstedt.

Libæk, I. 2000. 'Ett Nobelinstitutt eller 'Revue Nobel'? Konfliker i den første Nobelkom-miteen', *Det Norske Nobelinstitutts Skriftserie* Vol. 1 – No. 1. Oslo: Norwegian Nobel Institute.

Källstrand, G. 2012. *Medaljens framsida: Nobelpriset i pressen 1897–1911*. Stockholm: Carlsson.

Liljestrand, G. 1960. *Karolinska mediko-kirurgiska institutets historia 1910–1960* (2). Stockholm: Almqvist & Wicksell.

Lindqvist, S. 2011. 'The Nobel Prize as a Mirror of 20th-Century Science and Culture'. In *Changes in the technological landscape: Essays in the History of Science and Technol-ogy*, edited by Svante Lindqvist. Sagamore Beach: Science History Publications.

Lovell, L. 2006. *The Politics of Cultural Capital: China's Quest for a Nobel Prize in Litera-ture*. Honolulu: University of Hawai'i Press.

Luttenberger, F. 1997. *Nobelpriset som en vetenskaplig resurs: Diskussioner om ett medi-cinskt Nobelinstitut 1917–1922*. Uppsala: Avdelningen för vetenskapshistoria.

Rydén, P. 2011. *Den framgångsrike förloraren: En värderingsbiografi över Carl David af Wirsén*. Stockholm: Carlsson.

Sohlman, R. 1950. *Ett testamente: Hur Alfred Nobels dröm blev verklighet*. Stockholm: Atlantis.

Sörenson, U. 1992. *Ferdinand Boberg: Arkitekten som konstnär*. Höganäs: Wiken.

Urde, M. and Greyser, S.A. 2015. 'The Nobel Prize: the Identity of a Corporate Heritage Brand'. *Journal of Product and Brand Management Research* 24:4, 318–332.

Weinberg, A.M. 1961. 'Impact of large-scale science on the United States'. *Science* 134 (3473): 161–164.

Widmalm, S. 1995. 'Science and Neutrality: The Nobel Prizes of 1919 and Scientific Internationalism in Sweden'. *Minerva* 33:339–360.

Widmalm, S. 2012. 'A superior type of universal civilisation': Science as Politics in Sweden, 1917–1926'. In Rebecka Lettevall, Geert Somsen & Sven Widmalm (eds.), *Neutrality in Twentieth-Century Europe: Intersections of Science, Culture, and Politics after the First World War*. 65–89. London: Routledge.

CHAPTER 3

Hitler's Boycott: Cultural Politics and the Rhetoric of Neutrality

Sven Widmalm

The status of the Nobel Prize as the foremost international award in science was well established before the First World War.[1] It seemed to embody the fin-de-siècle dream of progress through friendly competition, manifested also in the large international expositions or the Olympic Games. During the war, its reputation was not exactly tarnished but as the general framework of the dream it had helped sustain collapsed, the prize became vulnerable to political interpretations casting doubt on the ideology that underpinned it: that such a thing as impartial judgement was possible, even in science, in a world rife with political conflict. The Nobel Prizes of 1919 were awarded against the background of international ostracism of Germany, also in science. The Swedish Academy of Sciences caused raised eyebrows when it awarded three Germans and no other nationals that year: Fritz Haber received the postponed 1918 chemistry prize (no 1919 chemistry prize was awarded); Max Planck received the postponed 1918 physics prize; Johannes Stark received the 1919 physics prize. There was no medicine prize awarded in 1919 though Jules Bordet would receive the postponed 1919 prize in 1920 (to make this even more confusing, the 1919 laureates would actually receive their awards in June 1920). Those who defended the academy claimed that it proved that it staunchly stood by ideals of impartiality, objectivity and neutrality. The terminology varied but the general idea was that the award decisions, like science itself, were a-political. Considering the fact that general suffrage, founded on party-political systems, was being introduced in many countries around this time (1919 in Sweden), the idea that science should be a-political, but that it maybe was not, resonated differently among different political fractions. In Sweden, right-wingers and some established scientists defended the Nobel Prizes of 1919 as logical from the perspective of scientific objectivity (the best scientists just happened to be German). The parliamentarian left (Social Democrats and Liberals) tended to consider them a demonstrative show of support for Germany or even German

---

1   Crawford 1984, Chapter 7.

militarism.[2] The notion of objective judgement, central not only to the idea that prestigious prizes should be fairly awarded but to the scientific enterprise as a whole, was thus politicized in connection with the 1919 Nobel awards.

The prestige of the Nobel Prize indeed makes it interesting to study from the perspective of science and politics, epistemology and ideology. Mostly this has been done from the points of view of media and of various power struggles within the relevant scientific specialties (physiology or medicine, physics, and chemistry).[3] This chapter has a slightly different take on the problem and focuses on science, politics and the Nobel Prize from the perspective of National Socialist cultural politics, an example of what has lately been called 'science diplomacy'. Like the controversy surrounding the Prizes of 1919, Hitler's boycott of all Nobel Prizes 1937–1945 illuminates the simultaneously political and scientific meaning of neutrality or impartiality, or objectivity – the three concepts are not easily distinguishable in the contexts that will be discussed here.[4]

Before looking closer at this episode a few words must be said about German cultural politics during the Third Reich.[5] First, science was included in cultural politics. Innovation or research policy had not been invented by those names in the interwar period; in countries like Sweden and Germany science was still very much seen as part of culture. Cultural politics – aiming to project a positive image of a country's culture abroad – evolved after the First World War in Germany and other European countries. Various schemes were devised to promote academic exchange; foundations like those named after Alexander von Humboldt and the Rockefeller family exemplify this kind of cultural politics. The Nobel Prize can be placed in the same category. The intention of Alfred Nobel seems to have been to promote international culture and science for the greater good of all, but in the process the Nobel Prize gave the Swedish scientific and literary establishments, and the Norwegian parliament, a central position in the distribution of international cultural capital, a vital resource in cultural politics.[6]

National Socialism departed from the norms established in the international system of academic exchange by making the objectives of the Nazi state a

---

2 Widmalm 1995; Friedman 2012.
3 Bucchi 2017; Källstrand 2012; Friedman 2001; Crawford 1984.
4 On this issue in a Swedish context, see several papers in Björkman, Lundell, Widmalm 2016. For an international context, see several papers in Lettevall, Somsen, Widmalm 2012.
5 On science policy and 'Kulturpolitik' in Nazi Germany, see for example Flachowsky 2008; Weiss 2005. For the cultural-political relations between Germany and Norway, similar to those in Sweden, see Karchen 2012, chapter 5. For discussions about this topic from a Swedish perspective, see Almgren 2005; Åkerlund 2010; Björkman, Lundell, Widmalm 2016.
6 On the cultural impact of the Nobel Prize, see Friedman 2001, Chapter 4; Källstrand 2012.

main goal in that every form of exchange was rigged and policed to ensure that it not only promoted national interests but also ideological conformity, so-called 'coordination' (*Gleichschaltung*). Cultural politics was indeed meant to have a high visibility, and no one was surprised that the German Ministry of Propaganda engaged in such activities. But coordination, racial persecution, and the promotion of alternatives to 'objective' Western science by e.g. Alfred Rosenberg and the SS made many wary or even hostile to academic exchange with Germany. Promotors of Nazi cultural politics, like the *Deutscher Akademischer Austauschdienst* (German Academic Exchange Service), therefore encouraged the scientific and scholarly exchange of renowned academics that were not seen as party ideologues. At the same time it was thought vital that Germans going abroad and foreigners visiting Germany should not be openly critical of the Hitler regime. Cultural politics in the Nazi state was therefore conducted partly under a cloak of secrecy, through the means of furtive diplomacy, including the use of informants. Hitler's decision to boycott the Nobel Prize brought the contradictions of Nazi cultural politics out into the open.[7] In Sweden, it was met with glee and scorn from the anti-fascists and with confusion from those who contemporaries labelled 'pro-German' – a euphemism, endorsed by the Nazis for those who were optimistic concerning developments in the 'new Germany'.[8] As we will see in the following two sections, members of the Nobel establishment in literature as well as science employed various 'diplomatic' strategies to convince Hitler to revoke the boycott, albeit without success.

Fredrik Böök and the 'pro-German' Reactions to the Boycott

When Hitler announced on January 30, 1937, that Germans would no longer be allowed to accept Nobel Prizes, the Swedish journalist and historian of literature Fredrik Böök was in Berlin. The boycott concerned him personally because he was a member of the Nobel Committee of the Swedish Academy (of literature) and was also known as an occasional apologist for the Hitler regime. A few years earlier he had given the following self-characteristic: 'An old liberal who pleads the attenuating circumstances of Nazism'.[9] Böök's biographer, Svante Nordin, has described his reaction to the boycott, published in the

---

7   Crawford 2000; Almgren 2017.
8   Almgren 2005.
9   Böök, quoted in: Nordin 1994, 306.

broadsheet *Svenska Dagbladet*, as a 'harsh attack against Hitler's decision'.[10] But Böök's position was more equivocal than what Nordin suggests.

The official reason for the boycott was that in 1936 the Norwegian Parliament had awarded the pacifist journalist Carl von Ossietzky the 1935 peace prize. The choice was controversial. Ossietzky had been convicted of treason during the Weimar period because he published information about German rearmaments violating the Versailles Treaty. He had served his sentence but, as a known anti-Nazi, was interned again in connection with the purges after the Reichstag fire in February 1933. He would die in a prison hospital in 1938 without having received the prize money.

The prize to Ossietzky was controversial outside Germany as well, not least in Norway and Sweden.[11] Böök's article about the Nobel Prize boycott is largely about the journalist who had 'betrayed his fatherland' and about the despicable Norwegians who had 'put their office into disrepute'.[12] He described the award as part of an anti-German campaign; Hitler's reaction was to some extent understandable because no 'German patriot can avoid stamping Ossietzky as a madman and a traitor'.[13] In Sweden, however, the boycott fomented a growing enmity towards the 'new Germany'. The many Swedish friends of Germany, who above all sought 'objectivity and impartiality', felt let down. One had endorsed at least some aspects of Hitler's policies, but this loyalty was now rewarded with spite, which was hurtful: 'For we are not made out of wood', Böök exclaimed rather pathetically.[14]

Böök blamed the decision to boycott the Nobel Prizes awarded in Sweden (the three science prizes and literature) on political 'fanaticism' but also claimed that it was based on a misunderstanding, an inability of the German public to distinguish between the different prizes. He had retrieved this explanation directly from the Ministry of Propaganda and Public Enlightenment, where he discussed the issue with the head of the press department, Alfred-Ingemar Berndt, in the beginning of February. In the eyes of Germans, Berndt said, the 'name of the Nobel prize' was forever tarnished. Berndt gave an account of this meeting that indicated that Böök had argued against the boycott in a way that we recognize from his newspaper article. He had stressed that it was perceived very negatively in 'pro-German' circles in Sweden and that it would contribute to Germany's cultural isolation. To Berndt he also

---

10   Böök, quoted in: Nordin 1994, 308.
11   Thue 1994.
12   Böök 1937.
13   Böök 1937.
14   Böök 1937.

said that the Swedish prize committees could never compromise on their mission and, if the leading candidate happened to be German, award the 'second best'.[15] In view of the hypersensitivity of the regime it is likely true, as Nordin writes, that Böök for a while became persona non grata in Berlin. But this soon changed, and Böök was pleased to note that Hermann Göring, in a personal audience, agreed with him that Hitler's decision was ill advised.[16] It was however not revoked.

Böök's reaction exemplifies some characteristic elements of the rhetoric of 'pro-German' intellectuals in Sweden. The traditional admiration of German culture and science was for example translated into respect for the National Socialist revolution. Böök and those similarly minded tended to explain criticism of the Hitler regime by a regrettable lack of sympathy for the special situation in Germany brought on by numerous disasters, not least Versailles. They underscored the need for objectivity, impartiality and neutrality – principles that were considered absent in the anti-German Swedish press. Such reasoning lay behind the foundation in 1937 of the Lund-based National Association Sweden-Germany (*Riksföreningen Sverige-Tyskland*) – perhaps the most important Swedish propaganda organization for the German cause throughout the Nazi era. Böök was not a member but some of his pro-German writings were published by the Association and adhered to the general rhetorical pattern of other writings promoted by the Association.[17]

This was indeed true of Böök's most notorious publication on Nazi Germany, an extended version of a talk given to students at Lund University in 1940 and published by the Association as a pamphlet and also as a book chapter (1940, 1941). Böök interpreted the implications of neutrality in the light of a presumed new European order with Germany as dominant power.[18] He was opposed to the idea that Sweden should become part of a Greater Germany; in his own way he supported a politics of neutrality. The neutral position corresponded to the Swedish essence, he said – it was logical considering the nation's historical experience. But neutrality also meant that the Nazi

---

15 Alfred-Ingemar Berndt, 'Aufzeichnung für Herrn Staatssekretär Dr. Lammers', Bundesarchiv Berlin-Lichterfelde, R 43 III/910 b. The document, written to the head of the Reich Chancellery Hans Heinrich Lammers, is an account of the conversation between Berndt and Böök. An accompanying letter is dated 6 February 1937 so the meeting should have taken place between 31 January and this date. From the letter, it is clear that Hitler had been told about the conversation and had said that he would inform the Swedish Government regarding his views.

16 Nordin 1994, 308–309.

17 Lundell 2016; Nordin 1994, 308–309.

18 Forser 1976, Chapter 13.

dictatorship – an undesirable, yet logical consequence of Germany's historical experience – must be treated with respect:

> How could you count on goodwill, if you do not give goodwill in re-turn? How could you ask for understanding, respect for Swedish essence and Swedish values, if you can not show understanding and sympathy for German essence, esteem and respect for German values? If we are mastered by the mentality created by the hatred of Germany during the world war and that, in the current crisis, is flourishing again, if we allow public opinion to be bullied and systematically poisoned by rabid party hacks, then our future is dark. Heavy clouds are gathering, and the storm becomes inevitable.[19]

The quote exemplifies Böök's rhetorical technique. He attributed criticism of the new Germany to sentiments deriving from anti-German feelings dur-ing the First World War rather than the Nazi period; thus anti-Nazism was a symptom of general hostility to Germany. Critics of Nazi Germany were 'rabid party hacks' – a typical example of how anti-democratic and pro-Nazi rhetoric worked. Neutrality, impartiality and objectivity were contrasted with the tyr-anny of special interest; realism was opposed to a defective 'sense of reality'.[20] A *rhetoric of neutrality*, in which Nazi critics were depicted as non-neutral, par-tisan or party political was characteristic of Böök's pamphlet, as well as other publications of the National Association Sweden-Germany.

Böök could be perceived as opportunistic: 'I think he rushes a bit as the wind blows', commented Astrid Lindgren.[21] Nordin rejects such an interpreta-tion on psychological grounds, and it does indeed not appear to be particularly useful from an analytical perspective. It can be said, however, that the posi-tion of Böök and likeminded was situation-dependent and that their writings were ideologically coordinated. Böök's pamphlet was an expression of a gen-eral 'pro-German' mindset in the autumn of 1940, which also saw the publi-cation of writings such as the radical right-wing youth call 'The Swedish line' (*Den svenska linjen*) by a group of young intellectuals, some of whom would become influential intellectuals after the war.[22] They too argued that Sweden must adapt to Nazi-ruled European order, as did the renowned law professor Karl Olivecrona's 'England or Germany', also published in the fall of 1940 and

---

19   Böök 1940, 47–48.
20   Böök 1940, 45.
21   Lindgren 2014, 70.
22   Larsmo 2016.

translated to many European languages. Olivecrona too argued, from a kind of legal-realistic view of neutrality and without even mentioning Nazism, in favour of a European order under German leadership. Hence Böök participated with like-minded intellectuals in the design of a rhetoric of neutrality that simultaneously claimed independence for the Swedish nation and proposed adaptation to a Nazi-led Europe.

The response to the boycott of the Nobel Prize should, when it comes to 'pro-German' Swedish intellectuals, be understood in such a context. The cultural union between the two Germanic peoples was threatened by the fact that the Führer distanced himself from the Nobel Prize, which had so often been awarded to Germans, for many years serving to strengthen ties between the two countries. The implicit questioning of the impartiality of the Swedish Nobel-awarding institutions became a wrench in the rhetorical machinery of 'pro-German' academics. 'To mighty Germany', Böök wrote, 'it may be a small matter [...], but there is a saying that you should not despise small wounds or poor friends'.[23] A few months later, Hitler poured salt into the wounds of his poor friends in Sweden by making the party ideologue Alfred Rosenberg and the Berlin surgeons Ferdinand Sauerbruch and August Bier, among others, the first recipients of the new national prize for art and science, instituted as a replacement for the Nobel Prize and only awarded to Germans![24]

Hans von Euler's Science Diplomacy

In discussions about Swedish academics that supported the new Germany, some names almost always appear. In addition to Böök, the explorer and writer Sven Hedin, the theologian Hugo Odeberg, the historian Gottfrid Carlsson, the race biologist Herman Lundborg, the geneticist Herman Nilsson-Ehle and Karl Olivecrona are usually mentioned. However, the number of 'pro German' intellectuals was significantly larger than those who took as clear a public stance as those just mentioned. One central figure was the chemist Hans von Euler-Chelpin. He had a leading position in Swedish-German circles and was (together with his friend Hedin) among the most important scientists outside of Germany supporting the Nazi regime. He was of German origin but a Swedish citizen and since 1929 a Nobel Prize Laureate in chemistry. During the interwar period, Euler was a central figure in Swedish science. Many rewards and honours, such as the Goethe Medal of Arts and Sciences and the election to

---

23   Böök 1937.
24   Hansson/Schagen 2014; Hansson 2015.

academies and similar associations, testify to his strong position in the Third Reich.[25]

In the sources concerning 'pro-German' Swedish academics, Euler is constantly present but always, it seems, careful not to take an explicit political stance. There is however no doubt that he was a central figure in these circles and that he was seen as such by contemporaries. In 1937, when he became chairman of the so-called German Colony in Stockholm (an umbrella organization for organizations that in various ways promoted Swedish-German relations), he was singled out by the leading liberal broadsheet *Dagens Nyheter* as a potential traitor. The paper claimed that the Colony was a 'Nazi Germany [...] outside of the country's borders [...] directly under the leadership of the Berlin Government' and that Euler, a Swedish citizen, was therefore 'in the service of a foreign power'.[26] Euler responded by claiming that the Colony was completely independent, which was hardly the case.[27] The Swedish security police kept an eye on the Colony and its reports show that the organization under Euler's leadership was thoroughly Nazified.[28] So for example, the organization arranged a meeting with the mayor of Berlin Julius Lippert as guest of honour and main speaker shortly after Euler had been elected chairman. Lippert was not just any Nazi official: he was a rabid anti-Semite, a former editor of *Der Angriff*, and (according to himself) a complicit in the murder of Walther Rathenau. He was introduced by the Colony's vice chairman Sven Hedin and gave a much appreciated talk on the enormous progress made in the German capital after 1933. When visiting Stockholm he not only spoke at the Colony but was honoured with a lunch with representatives of the Swedish Foreign Ministry (Euler participated as well) and was wined and dined by Hedin.[29] In January 1938 the Colony celebrated the fifth anniversary of the *Machtergreifung*. According to *Dagens Nyheter*, the Nazi eugenicist Arthur Gütt gave a speech and the envoy Wied 'led the audience in a fourfold Sieg Heil to the Third Reich and Adolf Hitler'.[30] It is quite clear that the organization that Euler led was an important bridgehead in Sweden for Nazi cultural politics. It is logical that diplomat Sven Grafström wrote, in connection with the German attacks on Norway and Denmark in April 1940, that 'local Quisslings [sic]' like Euler had reason to

---

25   Widmalm 2011.

26   Dagens Nyheter 1937a.

27   In response to Euler, the newspaper quoted new laws that concerned the 'coordination' of all German expats, implying that Euler simply lied (Dagens Nyheter 1937b).

28   Archives of the security police (*Säkerhetspolisens arkiv*) at The Swedish National Archives (*Riksarkivet*), F5 DD.

29   Dagens Nyheter 1937c; Dagens Nyheter 1937d.

30   Dagens Nyheter 1938.

worry about the security police taking action against them (Grafström 1989, 228). The professor of medicine Israel Holmgren – an anti-Nazi activist – reported Euler as well as Hedin to the police as potential 'traitors'. Euler's telephone was wiretapped for six weeks but nothing more incriminating than evidence of a 'pro German' attitude came to light.[31]

As a Nobel Laureate and a long-standing member of the Nobel Committee for Chemistry, Euler, like Böök in literature, saw himself as a guardian of the prize's status which he thought rested on ideals such as internationalism, objectivity and impartiality.[32] As we have seen, the prize's impartiality had been seriously questioned in 1919, when the Academy of Sciences gave the first three science prizes after the war to three Germans. The decision was defended by researchers from the Central Powers and by some Swedes as objective precisely because it *was* controversial, thus demonstrating that the prize was above politics.[33] Another type of crisis occurred twenty years later, again due to the award of three German researchers: the chemists Adolf Butenandt and Richard Kuhn, both with Euler as prime advocate in the Nobel Committee, and the bacteriologist Gerhard Domagk. The background was, of course, that the boycott against the prize was still in effect. We will now look more closely at the reactions in the Swedish scientific community when the boycott was first proclaimed and then discuss what happened when the three Germans were awarded.[34]

Dejection struck many Swedish researchers when Hitler's decision was made public. The Nobel Prize's international standing was threatened when Germany – the most Nobel-prize awarded nation in science and medicine – would no longer recognize its value.[35] Like Böök, Euler met with Göring, trying to make him change Hitler's mind (they knew each other since they had both been fighter pilots in Germany during the war).[36] But this led nowhere. A similar attempt by the physician Folke Henschen, who had family connections

---

31   Israel Holmgren, copies of two letters to the security police, 16 April 1940, Archives of the security police at The Swedish National Archives, files on individuals (*personakter*), Euler and Hedin. About the wiretapping, see Max Paulin, 'P-M. till ärende Hd.-2675/40', 5 July 1940, Euler's file.

32   Crawford 1984.

33   Widmalm 1995.

34   About Euler's support for the two chemistry Laureates, see Crawford 2000, 43; Friedman 2001, 202–203.

35   Nobel statistics was a recurring theme when the boycott was discussed. E.g. Hedin 1937, 257–258, and articles in Dagens Nyheter 1937e.

36   von Euler-Chelpin 1969, 134. There are copies of this manuscript at many Swedish university libraries, e.g. at Uppsala and the Karolinska Institute.

with Göring, did not give any results either.[37] After the boycott had come into effect, the Nobel establishment in Stockholm had to find a more long-term strategy to minimize its impact. Euler, who was a friend of the German Envoy in Stockholm, Victor, Prinz zu Wied, was to play a central role in the diplomatic exchanges that followed.

Wied made a survey of opinions regarding the boycott in Swedish newspapers and informed Berlin that these were almost exclusively negative: 'pro Germans' described it as an unforced error whereas anti-Nazis pointed out that the German intellectual elite was in exile anyhow, so that it would not have much of an effect.[38] In general, the boycott was interpreted in the context of German cultural politics, which was particularly sensitive to the common criticism that German science and culture were undermined by the Nazis' anti-science ideology and by the persecution of Jewish and other intellectuals.[39] Swedish 'pro Germans' deplored that the boycott strengthened the view that Nazi policies were disastrous for science and culture whereas critics of the regime saw it as a not very interesting confirmation of a well-established fact.

In at least one case the boycott met with public sympathy, namely from Sven Hedin – world famous 'explorer' and writer, friend of Euler as well as Böök, and a member of both Swedish Nobel-awarding academies. His comments in *Dagens Nyheter* were considered important enough to be communicated to Berlin almost verbatim, possibly because he was one of Hitler's favourite authors and was thought to have a special influence with the Führer, whom he met on a number of occasions.[40] Hedin agreed with Böök that Ossietzky was indeed a criminal who did not deserve any awards. He regretted that the Nobel Prize awarding institutions that, during 36 years 'in choosing laureates have shown an objectivity, a demand for justice, and a scrupulous impartiality that has never failed the responsibility entrusted in them' would suffer because of the wrongheadedness of the Norwegians. According to Hedin they had turned the peace prize into a 'party reward'; in the future it should be awarded in Sweden by 'Swedish men of whose impartiality and objectivity there can be no doubt, whatever party they belong to'.[41]

Euler and Wied discussed the situation immediately after the boycott was announced and the envoy then forwarded his friend's views to the German

37   Crawford 2000, 44.
38   Telegram from Wied to Auswärtiges Amt (AA), 31 January 1937, Auswärtiges Amt, Politisches Archiv, Stockholm (AAPS) 627; Wied to AA, 1 and 8 February 1937, ibid.
39   Widmalm 2016a.
40   Odelberg 2012.
41   S. Hedin, 'Hedin om Hitlers Nobelbeslut: Låt svenskar ge fredspriset', 1 February 1937, 1, 7. This article is described in detail in a letter from Wied to AA, 1 February 1937, AAPS 627.

Ministry of Foreign Affairs. Euler warned that the result could be more awards to German 'emigrants' (Jews, dissidents, and other undesirables in exile). This could have 'the unwelcome consequence' that they would have better economic opportunities to engage in the 'international struggle against Germany'. Moreover, it would become more difficult to claim that 'German science is capable of performing at a very high level, also without emigrant elements'. Euler's point was that Germany's friends in Sweden really did not want the cleansing of Jews and others to be regarded as a loss for German science. Implicitly Euler described the boycott as a direct threat against the objectives of Nazi cultural politics. In addition, the boycott could have serious economic consequences. In Sweden, the Nobel Prize was part of national identity, wrote Euler, and the Nobel Day (December 10, when the award ceremony took place) was a kind of National Day. Among the leadership of the Nobel Foundation, there were influential people from the business community who had been kindly disposed towards Germany but who were now bitterly disappointed.[42]

During the spring of 1937, the diplomatic stakes were raised as Hitler decreed that the regime would see it as a hostile act when Germans were awarded with Nobel Prizes. In April, Foreign Minister Constantin von Neurath called on Wied telling him to ask Euler if it was possible to prevent this from happening.[43] Euler stuck to the official line and rejected the idea that the price-awarding institutions would be influenced by the boycott: the prize-awarding institutions would take only scientific or literary merit into account.[44] As far as the three scientific Nobel Committees were concerned, only 'exclusively objective scientific criteria' counted. The Swedish Nobel Prizes must not be suspected of the same bias as the Peace Prize.[45] The general opinion among 'pro-German' researchers in Sweden was, according to Euler, that Germany's cause was best helped by awarding prizes to the country's great scientists! If this were no longer possible, 'the less German-minded gentlemen' would take advantage of the opportunity to award 'other nations and races'. The letter ended with both 'Heil Hitler!' and 'deutscher Gruss' (German greeting).

In September 1939, Euler let it be known to the Germans that proposals had been made to award a Nobel Prize in medicine to an 'Aryan Reich-German' and two in chemistry to Germans, of which one was an Nazi-party member and the

---

42   Wied, 'Aufzeichnung', 5 February 1937. This is a description of Euler's views. Another version, where Euler's name is not mentioned, was sent to AA, 9 February 1937. Both documents are in AAPS 627. The quotes here are from the first version where Euler is named.

43   Constantin von Neurath to Wied, 12 April 1937, AAPS 627.

44   The official line was expressed e.g. in the following news articles: Dagens Nyheter 1937f; Dagens Nyheter 1937g; Dagens Nyheter 1939.

45   Wied to von Neurath, 5 May 1937; Euler to Wied, 3 May 1937. Both letters are in AAPS 627.

other President of the German Chemistry Society. Good choices all three from a Nazi perspective, one would think. Euler pointed out that the prizes should be seen as an 'impartial recognition' of German science and that this was particularly 'noteworthy at a time when Germany is waging war'.[46] This was obviously correct (there were no other Laureates from warring nations that year). The comment mirrored the rhetoric used to defend the 1919 Nobel Prizes: they should be seen as particularly objective because they were awarded in a situation when political opinion might react negatively to such a one-sided decision, not least from neutral Sweden.

In case Euler believed that Hitler would appreciate the three Nobel Prizes, he was mistaken. In November, Wied was recalled to Berlin for consultation. Before this minor diplomatic crisis broke out, the new Foreign Minister, Joachim von Ribbentrop, had made an attempt to give the incident more serious diplomatic proportions. He suggested that the prizes could be accepted after all, if the money could be donated to a Swedish National Socialist organization, and he asked Wied to investigate if there were any suitable candidates.[47] Wied said that two such organizations existed but that both were committed to maintaining a strictly national line and that they would therefore probably reject a proposal that would make them appear as German puppets.[48] Two days later came the formal diplomatic protest where Ribbentrop completely rejected the idea that Nobel-Prize decisions at the Karolinska Institute and the Academy of Sciences were 'formally independent'. It was, he wrote, unthinkable that these institutions could ignore a 'serious' prompting from the Government.[49] Hence Ribbentrop demonstratively dismissed the hallowed notion that the Nobel Prize-awarding institutions were independent and impartial. The seriousness of the regime's position on this issue was made clear when the medicine laureate, Gerhard Domagk (awarded for the anti-bacterial drug prontosil) unwisely sent a letter of thanks to the Karolinska Institute and was promptly arrested by the Gestapo. Domagk was not a Nazi but nevertheless a collaborator of the regime; thanks to the overreaction of the Gestapo he would however receive a hero's welcome when he was finally able to come to Stockholm and receive his award (but no money) in 1947.[50]

---

46   Euler to Wied, 27 September 1939. An almost verbatim account of Euler's views were sent by Wied to AA two days later. Both letters are at AAPS 627.

47   Werner von Grundherr to Wied, 16 November 1939, AAPS 627.

48   Wied to AA, 16 November 1939, AAPS 627.

49   Joachim von Ribbentrop to Wied (including an 'Aide-Memoire' to the Swedish Foreign Minister Rickard Sandler), 18 November 1939, AAPS 627.

50   Crawford 2000; Almgren 2017. On the effects of the boycott on medicine in general, see Hansson 2015; Hansson and Schagen 2014.

The 'Jewish Question'

Like Böök and others, Euler had failed to influence the regime in Germany. This was despite the fact that he had aligned himself closely with Nazi ideology when arguing against the boycott, e.g. by pointing to the threat constituted by 'emigrants' and 'other races' being awarded instead. Officially the boycott did not have anything to do with the 'Jewish question', but contemporaries nevertheless did make this connection. According to the Berlin correspondent of *Dagens Nyheter*, the newly established 'Research Institute for the Jewish Question' in Munich had initiated an investigation of the racial descent of the Nobel Committee and of Nobel Laureates, and also of the Nobel Committee members' views of the 'Jewish question'.[51] According to the newspaper, several Swedish researchers had received questions concerning such matters from Munich.[52] *Dagens Nyheter* speculated that the boycott was, in fact, an attack on the cosmopolitan ideology represented by the Nobel Prize and regarded by the Nazis as a typical Jewish phenomenon.[53]

In many ways this interpretation is plausible. An indication is that the boycott was announced when anti-Semitic so-called German (or Aryan) physics, led by Nobel Laureates Johannes Stark and Philipp Lenard, launched an offensive against the kind of theoretical physics that had been awarded a series of Nobel Prizes in the years after the First World War. Lenard, who, according to *Dagens Nyheter*, was behind the letters concerning Jewish Nobel Laureates, had just published his four volume work on 'German Physics', and Stark would soon endorse the denunciation of the leading theorist Werner Heisenberg as a 'White Jew' and 'the Ossietzky of Physics' by the SS journal *Das Schwarze Korps*.[54] In November 1936, the 'Research Institute for the Jewish Question' in Munich arranged a meeting, the proceedings of which were published in the first volume of its yearbook. Lenard contributed a short paper emphasizing the negative impact of the Nobel Prize on German science after the war (Lenard 1937, 41–44). Awards to the likes of Albert Einstein and Niels Bohr had strengthened the position of abstract and subjective Jewish science at the expense of realistic and objective Aryan science. Joseph Goebbels noted, also in November 1936, that Hitler wanted to connect the planned boycott with the greater

---

51   About the institute, see Berg 2008.
52   Dagens Nyheter 1937h.
53   Dagens Nyheter 1937f.
54   Relevant documents are translated in Hentschel 1996, 152–160; Walker 1995, Chapter 2.

issue of foreign awards in the context of a 'general attack on world Jewry' (28. November 1936).[55]

There is no direct evidence that Euler was aware of anti-Semitic intentions behind the boycott. An indication, besides that he used anti-Semitic arguments against the boycott, is that he and Hedin discussed Jewish Nobel Prize winners a few weeks before the boycott was proclaimed.[56] This may have been because of a request from the Munich Institute or other indications that the prize was perceived as problematic from an anti-Semitic point of view. According to Euler's autobiography, he became aware of the planned boycotts already in 1935, which may indicate that the Ossietzky affair was a triggering factor behind an anti-Semitically motivated decision.[57]

Soul Searching

The interpretation of the 'pro-German' rhetoric concerns moral questions on several levels: how should the historian determine what kind of actions were reasonable in relation to the Third Reich, and what is the measure of reasonability, then or now? It is necessary to dig as deeply as possible, even though definitive answers may not be found. Magnus Alkarp discovered from such an historical excavation that the archaeologist Sune Lindqvist, who seemingly belonged to the pro-Nazi camp in Sweden, in fact collaborated with the security police to counter German infiltration, and that he was an active anti-Nazi also in other respects.[58] In Lindqvist's case appearances deceived.

What about Böök and Euler? The former appeared sometimes as a supporter of the Hitler regime and at other times as a critic. By contemporaries he was not definitely placed in the Nazi camp until he made the infamous speech, mentioned above, at Lund University in 1940.[59] After the war, Böök himself raised the issue of guilt. In the autobiographical book *Rannsakan* ('Soul searching') he compared Nazi genocide, Soviet slave camps, the Allied terror bombings

---

55   Goebbels and Frölich (ed.) 2001, 267.
56   Euler to Hedin, 14 January 1937, Hedin's papers, The Swedish National Archives (used by permission). The letter contains, with reference to a conversation the previous day, a list of Jewish Nobel Laureates in science and medicine.
57   Crawford 2000, 38. According to the journalist Hertha Pauli, members of the Board of the Nobel Foundation corroborated that the boycott had an anti-Semitic background (Pauli 1945, 21). Pauli was the sister of Wolfgang Pauli who received his Nobel Prize in the same month that her article was printed.
58   Alkarp 2009, 345–354.
59   Nordin 1994, 321–325.

in Germany, and the use of nuclear weapons in Japan.[60] According to Böök, all these horrors were still (in 1953!) defended by some. He concluded that the only thing the horrors of the Second World War taught us was that all men are sinful, 'all without exception, and first and foremost ourselves'.[61] According to historian of literature Ture Stenström this showed that Böök 'in pious naivety sought to accept and understand even Nazi violence'.[62] But the view that wickedness was evenly distributed between dictatorships and democracies should perhaps be interpreted as yet another variation of the rhetoric of neutrality.

As for Euler, the sources are limited with respect to his political or ideological views. He often figures in the exchange of information between German Legation in Stockholm and the Foreign Ministry in Berlin, always described as politically reliable. In 1939, when Berlin wanted information about Swedish researchers invited to Vienna, the envoy Wied for example wrote that Euler was a personal friend of Göring's and completely dedicated to the German cause.[63] Evidence that Euler, as the diplomat Sven Grafström suggested, was a potential fifth columnist is provided in his unpublished autobiography, written in the early 1960s. It lacks self-awareness and consists mostly of reports of scientific work and foreign contacts. The many journeys Euler made to Germany during the Nazi era, and the many honours he received from the German research community and from the regime, are mechanically listed. Euler neither justified nor defended his close association with Hitler Germany. The only important indication in this regard is an annoyed remark to the effect that he received Jewish researchers at his laboratory which showed that he was not anti-Semitic. Euler did comment that the Nazi establishment was partly composed of impractical and incompetent types, but there is no evidence that he re-evaluated his collaboration with the regime.[64]

In individual cases like these, historical analyses often cannot lead to conclusions that are unequivocal. Technically speaking Böök and Euler were not Nazis, and by and large they probably did not sympathize with the extreme aspects of Nazi ideology; both (especially Böök) spoke out against the persecution of Jews but sometimes also adopted anti-Semitic rhetoric. We may call them fellow travellers ('Mitläufer') – a rather neutral term that refers to certain types of actions rather than underlying beliefs. More informative is to use this duo and like-minded colleagues as historical raw material in the study of movements

---

60   Böök 1953.
61   Böök 1953; Björklund 2004.
62   Stenström 1976, 152.
63   Wied to AA, 28 February 1939, 'Betreff: Vorträge schwedischer Wissenschaftler in Wien', AAPS 339.
64   Widmalm 2011.

and dislocations in academic culture during a time when democracy and scientific liberty were put under serious threat. Posterity's verdict concerning the adaptability of German academic culture to the Hitler regime has been harsh. The supposedly neutral Swedish 'pro-Germans' apparently made preparations, from a convenient distance, to effect a similar adaptation – as Böök put it, to join 'a European Völkergemeinschaft [...], where the Nordic people are closest to the centre'.[65]

Claiming to represent an ideal of impartiality, 'pro-German' Swedish intellectuals like Böök and Euler seemed to endorse the Hitler regime. The rhetoric of neutrality might seem like a smoke screen behind which Nazi interests were promoted. But it could also be seen as an attempt to protect Swedish interests or the status of the Nobel Prize. Either way, it suggests the highly political nature of the rhetoric of 'neutrality' or 'objectivity' surrounding the Nobel Prize.

This chapter is an extended version of a paper published in Swedish: Widmalm 2016b.

Bibliography

Åkerlund, A. 2010. *Mellan akademi och kulturpolitik: Lektorat i svenska språket vid tyska universitet 1906–1945*. Uppsala: Acta Universitatis Upsaliensia.

Alkarp, M. 2009. *Det Gamla Uppsala: Berättelser & metamorfoser*. Uppsala: Institutionen för arkeologi och antik historia.

Almgren, B. 2005. *Drömmen om Norden: Nazistisk infiltration 1933–1945*. Stockholm: Carlssons.

Almgren, B. 2017. 'Der Nobelpreis – ehrenvolle wissenschaftliche Auszeichnung oder unfreundlicher Akt? Wissenschaft zwischen Integrität und Anpassung'. In *It's Dynamite – Der Nobelpreis im Wandel der Zeit*, edited by N. Hansson and T. Halling, 27–38. Göttingen: Cuvillier.

Berg, M. 2008. 'Forschungsabteilung Judenfrage des Reichsinstituts für Geschichte des neuen Deutschlands'. In *Handbuch der völkischen Wissenschaften*, edited by I. Haar and M. Fahlbusch, 168–178. München: K.G. Saur.

Björklund, S. 2004. 'Fredrik Böök på det sluttande planet'. *Scandia* 70 (1): 61–81.

Björkman, M.; Lundell, P.; Widmalm (ed.), S. 2016. *De intellektuellas förräderi? Relationer mellan Sverige och Tredje riket inom vetenskap och kultur*. Lund: Arkiv.

Böök, F. 1937. 'Nobelpriset och Tredje riket'. *Svenska Dagbladet*, 8 March 1937: p. 7–8.

Böök, F. 1940. *Tyskt väsen och svensk lösen*. Malmö: Dagens böcker.

Böök, F. 1953. *Rannsakan*. Stockholm: Bonniers.

---

65   Böök 1940, 54; Thulstrup 1941, 100–101.

Bucchi, M. 2017. *Come vincere un Nobel. Geni, eroi e santi: l'immagine pubblica della scienza*. Torino: Einaudi.

Crawford, E. 1984. *The Beginnings of the Nobel Institution: The Science Prizes, 1901–1915*. Cambridge: Cambridge University Press.

Crawford, E. 2000. 'German Scientists and Hitler's Vendetta against the Nobel Prize'. *Historical Studies in the Physical and Biological Sciences* 31(1): 37–53.

Dagens Nyheter. 1937a. 'Tyskar i Sverige'. 5 February: p. 3.

Dagens Nyheter. 1937b. 'Professor Euler förklarar sig'. 6 February: p. 3.

Dagens Nyheter. 1937c. 'Svensk-tyska'. 9 April: p. 14.

Dagens Nyheter. 1937d. 'Lunch för Lippert'. 10 April: p. 12.

Dagens Nyheter. 1937e. 'Tysk får ej ta emot Nobelpris' 31 January: p. 1.

Dagens Nyheter. 1937f. 'Nobelprisen'. 8 February: p. 3.

Dagens Nyheter. 1937g. 'Norsk tillfredsställelse över att tyskar prisbelönats'. 11 November: p. 17.

Dagens Nyheter. 1937h. 'Nobelintresse hos nazistisk 'naturvetenskap': Pristagarnas härstamning undersöks av institut i München'. 5 February: p. 4.

Dagens Nyheter. 1938. 'Femårsminnet'. 31 January: p. 12.

Dagens Nyheter. 1939. 'Pressgrannar'. 29 October: p. 4.

von Euler-Chelpin, H. 1969. *Minnen: Hans von Euler-Chelpin 1873–1964* (photo copy of manuscript, 1969).

Flachowsky, S. 2008. *Von der Notgemeinschaft zum Reichsforschungsrat: Wissenschaftspolitikim Kontext von Autarkie, Aufrüstung und Krieg*. Stuttgart: Franz Steiner Verlag.

Forser, T. 1976. *Bööks 30-tal: En studie i ideologi*. Stockholm: Pan.

Friedman, R.M. 2001. *The Politics of Excellence: Behind the Nobel Prizes in Science*. New York: W.H. Freeman.

Friedman, R.M. 2012. '"Has the Swedish Academy of Sciences ... seen nothing, heard nothing, and understood nothing?" The First World War, Biased Neutrality, and the Nobel Prizes in Science'. In *Neutrality in Twentieth-Century Europe: Intersections of Science, Culture, and Politics after the First World War*, edited by R. Lettevall, S. Widmalm, G. Somsen, 90–114. London and New York: Routledge.

Goebbels, J. and Frölich, E. (ed.). 2001. *Die Tagebücher von Joseph Goebbels*, Part I, Vol. 3:II. München: Saur.

Grafström, S. 1989. *Anteckningar 1938–1944*. Stockholm: Kungl. Samfundet för utgivande av handlingar rörande Skandinaviens historia.

Hansson, N. and Schagen, U. 2014. '"In Stockholm hatte man offenbar irgendwelche Gegenbewegung" – Ferdinand Sauerbruch (1875–1951) und der Nobelpreis'. *NTM* 22 (3): 133–161.

Hansson, N. 2015. '"Ein Umschwung des medizinischen Denkens" oder ,eine übereifrige literarische Tätigkeit'? August Bier, die Homöopathie und der Nobelpreis 1906–1936'. *Jahrbuch für Medizin, Gesellschaft, Geschichte* 33: 217–246.

Hedin, S. 1937. *Tyskland och världsfreden*. Stockholm: Medéns.

Hentschel, K. 1996. *Physics and National Socialism: An Anthology of Primary Sources*. Basel; Boston; Berlin: Birkhäuser Verlag.

Karchen, N.K. 2012. *Zwischen Nationalsozialismus und nordischer Gesinnung: Eine Studie zu den rechtsgerichteten Verbindungen norwegisch-deutscher Milieus in der Zwischenkriegszeit*. Oslo: Det humanistiske fakultet, Universitetet i Oslo.

Källstrand, G. 2012. *Medaljens framsida: Nobelpriset i pressen 1897–1911*. Stockholm: Carlssons.

Larsmo, O. 2016. 'Det svarta nätet: Om Unghögern, SNF och Sverigedemokraterna'. In *De intellektuellas förräderi? Relationer mellan Sverige och Tredje riket inom vetenskap och kultur*, edited by M. Björkman, P. Lundell and S. Widmalm, 307–336. Lund: Arkiv.

Lenard, P. 1937. 'Botschaft von Philipp Lenard', *Forschungen zur Judenfrage*. Hamburg: Hanseatische Verlagsanstalt Hamburg.

Lettevall, R.; Widmalm, S.; Somsen, G. 2012. *Neutrality in Twentieth-Century Europe: Intersections of Science, Culture, and Politics after the First World War*, edited by R. Lettevall, S. Widmalm, G. Somsen. London and New York: Routledge.

Lindgren, A. 2014. *Krigsdagböcker 1939–1945*. Stockholm: Salikon förlag.

Lundell, P. 2016. 'De välvilligas rationalitet: Objektivitetsideal och mediekritik inom Riksföreningen Sverige-Tyskland 1938 till 1958'. In *De intellektuellas förräderi? Relationer mellan Sverige och Tredje riket inom vetenskap och kultur*, edited by M. Björkman, P. Lundell and S. Widmalm, 277–306. Lund: Arkiv.

Nordin, S. 1994. *Fredrik Böök: En levnadsteckning*. Stockholm: Natur och Kultur.

Odelberg, A. 2012. *Vi som beundrade varandra så mycket: Sven Hedin och Adolf Hitler*. Stockholm: Norstedts.

Pauli, H. 1945. 'Nobel's Prizes and the Atom Bomb'. *Commentary Magazine* 1(2): 17–26.

Stenström, T. 1976. 'Fredrik Böök och nazismen'. In *Från Snoilsky till Sonnevi: Litteraturvetenskapliga studier tillägnade Gunnar Brandell*, edited by J. Stenkvist, 130–153. Stockholm: Natur och kultur.

Thue, E. 1994. *Nobels fredspris – og diplomatiske vorviklinger*. Oslo: Institutt for forsvarsstudier.

Thulstrup, Å. 1941. *Fredrik Böök som politisk skriftställare*. Stockholm: Wahlström och Widstrand.

Walker, M. 1995. *Nazi Science: Myth, Truth, and the German Atomic Bomb*. New York and London: Plenum Press.

Weiss, S.F. 2005. 'The Sword of Our Science' as a Foreign Policy Weapon: The Function of German Genetics in the International Arena during the Third Reich*. Berlin: Präsidentenkommission 'Geschichte der Kaiser-Wilhelm-Gesellschaft im Nationalsozialismus'.

Widmalm, S. 1995. 'Science and Neutrality: The Nobel Prizes of 1919 and Scientific Internationalism in Sweden'. *Minerva* 33: 339–360.

Widmalm, S. 2011. 'Selbstporträt eines Weggefährten. Hans von Euler-Chelpin und das Dritte Reich'. In *Fremde Wissenschaftler im Dritten Reich: Die Debye-Affäre im Kontext*, edited by D. Hoffmann and Mark Walker, 438–459. Göttingen: Wallstein Verlag.

Widmalm, S. 2016a. 'Vetenskap som propaganda: Akademiska kontakter mellan Sverige och Tyskland under Tredje riket'. In *De intellektuellas förräderi? Relationer mellan Sverige och Tredje riket inom vetenskap och kultur*, edited by M. Björkman, P. Lundell and S. Widmalm, 59–94. Lund: Arkiv.

Widmalm, S. 2016b. 'Nobelpriset och Tredje riket: Fredrik Böök, Hans von Euler och neutralitetens retorik'. In *Spänning och nyfikenhet: Festskrift till Johan Svedjedal*, edited by G. Furuland et al., 332–347. Möklinta: Gidlunds förlag.

PART 2

Laureates and Nominees

∵

From Global Recognition to Global Health: Antimicrobials and the Nobel Prize, 1901–2015

Scott H. Podolsky

This paper starts with a story about Bernard Lown, a world-renowned cardiologist at the Brigham and Women's Hospital, and one of the inventors of both cardiac defibrillation and the cardiac intensive care unit. He was likewise one of the co-founders of IPPNW, International Physicians for the Prevention of Nuclear War, for which he and his fellow co-founders would win the Nobel Peace Prize in 1985. As Lown humorously recalls, when the press phoned his mother to inform her of her son's Nobel Prize, she retorted, 'better he should have received a Nobel Prize in medicine'.[1] The lines between medicine and public health are quite fuzzy, and one could argue that IPPNW has saved far more lives than has the defibrillator or the intensive care unit. Nevertheless, over the past 118 years, the Nobel Prize selectors have seemed to know what they call 'medicine' and what they call 'peace', with the distinction based far more on means than ends.[2]

And with respect to the Nobel Prize in Physiology or Medicine itself, attention to the basic science of therapeutics and drug discovery has long seemed to overshadow attention to the *delivery* of those remedies to the populations who need them. I've had the chance to think about this often in recent years, as I have had the privilege of serving in a department with Paul Farmer and many of the clinician-researchers at Partners in Health, or PIH, which has justly received credit for bringing attention to the plight of the world's poorest populations, and to creating the infrastructure in countries like Haiti, Peru, and Rwanda for the delivery of sophisticated medical care that may rival what we deliver in Boston. But PIH, inspired by both the longer history

---

1 Lown 2008, 345.
2 The very first Nobel Peace Prize, in 1901, went to Henry Dunant for his role in the founding of the International Committee of the Red Cross. Subsequent awards have included the 1944 and 1963 awards to the International Committee of the Red Cross itself, the 1952 award to Albert Schweitzer for his medical work in Gabon, and the 1999 award to Médecins Sans Frontières. Two awards have gone to those improving global nutrition, the 1949 award to John Boyd Orr, and the 1970 award to Norman Borlaug.

© KONINKLIJKE BRILL NV, LEIDEN, 2019 | DOI:10.1163/9789004406421_006

of the use of community health workers in the delivery of care, as well as a liberation theology ethos emphasizing 'accompanying' those in need, has also advanced the use of community-based 'accompagnateurs' and social support in ensuring adherence to the complex regimens involved in the treatment of HIV, tuberculosis (TB), and multi-drug-resistant tuberculosis (MDR-TB).[3] Through the use of such accompagnateurs, they've been able to transform diseases perceived as untreatable – e.g., MDR-TB and extensively-drug resistant tuberculosis (XDR-TB) among the poorest inhabitants of Lima – into treatable diseases, serving as a paradigm for such possibility.[4] And as I teach about drug adherence and accompagnateurs each year, and likewise annually wonder if this is the year PIH will win the Nobel Peace Prize, I've found myself wondering: if accompaniment were found to improve adherence by a significant percentage, leading to significant changes in outcomes; and if it were found to make previously untreatable infections treatable, then shouldn't its proponents be eligible not only for the Nobel Peace Prize, but for the Nobel Prize in Physiology or Medicine as well? Perhaps yes, perhaps no, but these were the tensions I had in mind – between basic and applied science, medicine and public health, magic bullets and the structures in which they're embedded, and ultimately, between therapeutic means and ends – when I began constructing this chapter on the 118-year-old history of Nobel Prizes for antimicrobials.

I will thus use the history of the Nobel Prize for antimicrobials as a window on the history of antimicrobials more broadly, with certain Prizes serving as paradigms – or perhaps more appropriately, exemplars – for the treatment of infections for a series of foreseeable futures. These recursive futures themselves have performed important work, helping to mobilize support and funding for particular approaches to infectious diseases.[5] At the same, such a pattern of recursive – and often, over-optimistic – futures is itself somewhat humbling, in retrospect. I would then like to explore key underlying tensions exhibited across such a narrative, and perhaps most fundamentally, to examine the manner by which the Prizes have been presented and announced to the world, and thus their likely impact on our very faith in magic bullets themselves, and in our relative neglect of the delivery of such remedies to those who need them in the first place.

---

3   Farmer 2013.
4   Behforouz, Farmer, Mukherjee 2004; Shin, Furin, Bayona et al. 2004; Mitnick, Shin, Seung et al. 2008.
5   On the generative power of 'futures' in medical discourse, see Podolsky and Kveim Lie 2016.

Recursive Futures

Setting the contours of the discussion, it should be noted that out of the 109 Nobel Prizes in Physiology or Medicine, 28 have been devoted to infectious diseases or immunology. Of these, 11 have been devoted to immunology. And of the 17 devoted to infectious diseases, 6 have been explicitly awarded for antimicrobials per se, starting from the very beginning (see also Jacalyn Duffin's chapter in this volume). The Golden Age of Bacteriology of the 1870s and 1880s was almost immediately followed by the birth of immunology – including applied immunology, founded on the discovery and production of humoral antitoxins. And it is no accident that the very first Nobel Prize in Physiology or Medicine was awarded in 1901 to Emil von Behring for the development of diphtheria antiserum. Proven efficacious by one of the first controlled clinical studies, overcoming the skepticism that may have remained after the 1890s demise of its fellow proposed specific, Robert Koch's tuberculin treatment for tuberculosis, diphtheria antiserum, by 1901, appeared to serve at the vanguard of an expanding array of serotherapeutic remedies.[6] As Count Karl Mörner declared in his presentation speech: 'Up until now, serum therapy has had particularly splendid triumphs in the case of diphtheria, but its significance is not limited to this disease but extends much further. The field which is opened up for research by the development of serum therapy has therefore – for the present – no discernible limits'.[7] Indeed, the term 'magic bullet' itself was coined in 1906 by Paul Ehrlich to refer to serotherapy, to which chemotherapy could only aspire.[8] But despite the fact that proponents of serotherapy and active vaccine therapy received at least 230 nominations for the Nobel Prize in Physiology or Medicine between 1901 and 1940,[9] the future of serotherapy would be far more limited. Its most prominent representative, antipneumococcal antiserum, reflected both the possibilities and limitations of the remedy. Described in some quarters as a 'therapeutic revolution', and in others as 'the eugenic child of modern clinical medicine, representing the fruition of the mating of pure science with clinical medicine', antipneumococcal serotherapy became the focus

---

6 Hróbjartsson, Gøtzsche, Gludd 1998; Linton 2005.
7 Nobel Media AB 2014d.
8 Ehrlich 1906.
9 Data derived from Nobel Prize nomination database, at http://www.nobelprize.org/nomination/archive/ (accessed February 21, 2019). Approximately half of these nominations went to Émile Roux, who never did win the Prize. See also Luttenberger 1996. On the early dominance of bacteriology itself in the awarding of Nobel Prizes for Physiology or Medicine, see Salomon-Bayet 1982.

of coordinated national efforts against pneumonia in the United States and Denmark by the late 1930s.[10] But such serotherapy was only partially effective, logistically complicated, and expensive.

And it would soon be replaced and historically overshadowed by the long hoped-for antibacterial chemotherapeutic magic bullets, the dye-based sulfa drugs. They would be introduced by Gerhard Domagk in 1935, for which he would garner the Nobel Prize in 1939.[11] As John Lesch has described, the sulfa drugs appeared to practitioners and the public alike as 'miracle drugs', emblematic of the power of pharmaceutical research, and described in the language of conquest.[12] And once again, an expansive future was put forth, this time in the 1939 Nobel Prize presentation speech by the Karolinska Institute's Nanna Svartz:

> Whereas it proved possible to attack certain diseases due to protozoa and spirochetes by means of chemical substances [e.g., Ehrlich's own magic bullet, Salvarsan], little success had been achieved with chemical preparations against infections due to true bacteria, namely cocci and bacilli. The theory that bacteria of the last-mentioned categories could not be combated by chemical means therefore continued to gain ground, and it was consequently assumed that serotherapy was the most practicable method of treating infections of this type. ...[But now,] reports on the most brilliant therapeutic results with sulphonamide preparations are streaming in from all parts of the world. ...The imagination reels before the prospects of new chemotherapeutic victories which the sulphonamide preparations have unfolded before us.[13]

And in a follow-up presentation speech eight years later, despite increasing observations of sulfa drug resistance and toxicity, such expansiveness persisted: 'We can now justifiably believe that in the future infectious diseases will be eradicated by means of chemical compounds'.[14]

This last addendum seems an odd statement, as by that time, the industrially-derived sulfa drugs had already been superseded by perhaps the most iconic wonder drug of the 20th century, penicillin, for which Alexander Fleming, Howard Florey, and Ernst Chain had garnered the Prize in 1945, signaling that

---

10   Gray and Fulton 1938; Potts 1937; Podolsky 2006.

11   However, he would not receive the Prize in person until 1947, owing to Nazi interference – see Sven Widmalm's article in this volume, as well as Grundmann 2004.

12   Lesch 2007; Sherwood Taylor 1942.

13   Nobel Media AB 2014f.

14   Ibid.

'in a time when annihilation and destruction through the inventions of man have been greater than ever before in history, the introduction of penicillin is a brilliant demonstration that human genius is just as well able to save life and combat disease'.[15] Indeed, as Robert Bud has described, penicillin would serve as the focus of the re-branding of an increasingly powerful medical profession itself on both sides of the Atlantic in the post-War era.[16]

Mycologist Selman Waksman had coined the very term 'antibiotic' in 1942,[17] and he would propel forward what Fleming, in his Nobel Prize speech, termed 'intensive research into antibacterial products produced by moulds and other lowly members of the vegetable kingdom',[18] isolating streptomycin in 1943 and seemingly providing a cure for the original 'Captain of the Men of Death' and Koch's Bête noire, tuberculosis. By 1952, Waksman would earn the Nobel Prize, and Rutgers would prepare a media guidebook with the biblical nod that 'from the earth shall come salvation'.[19] And by then, soil-derived 'broad-spectrum' antibiotics like Aureomycin, Chloromycetin, and Terramycin served to exemplify the power of the medical and pharmaceutical professions to confront infectious diseases, leading to Nobelist Macfarlane Burnet's 1962 assessment, once again, that the twentieth century had witnessed 'the virtual elimination of the infectious diseases as a significant factor in social life'.[20]

By the 1980s, however, not only had antibiotic resistance and the AIDS epidemic tempered such enthusiasm, but the ideal of soil-sifting and screening had, in the context of diminishing returns, yielded to the notion of rational drug design.[21] Already in his Nobel Prize speech in 1945, Fleming had predicted that 'we are in a chemical age and penicillin may be changed by the chemists so that all its disadvantages may be removed and a newer and better derivative may be produced'.[22] And by 1988, Gertrude Elion and George Hitchings

---

15   Nobel Media AB 2014c.
16   Bud 2007.
17   Waksman 1973.
18   Fleming 1945, 92.
19   See Box 10, ff 33, Selman Waksman papers, Rutgers University. As has been discussed at length elsewhere, controversy would ensue over the relative contributions of Waksman and his graduate student, Albert Schatz, to the discovery of streptomycin in particular. See, e.g., Pringle 2012.
20   Podolsky 2015; Burnet 1962, 3; Later that decade, U.S. Surgeon General William H. Stewart is reported to have stated that 'it is time to close the book on infectious diseases, and declare the war against pestilence won', but the quote's sourcing remains elusive and it may well be apocryphal; see Spellberg 2008, 294.
21   As Arthur Daemmrich has described, at Pfizer this transition had already started by the 1960s; see Daemmrich 2009.
22   Fleming 1945, 92.

would garner the Prize (along with James Black) 'for their discoveries of important principles for drug treatment', as exemplified by their studies of nucleic acid metabolism that led not only to cancer chemotherapeutic agents like 6-mercaptopurine and azathioprine, but to such remedies as trimethoprim-sulfamethoxazole (sold as Septra or Bactrim) and acyclovir. As the Nobel Prize committee announced, 'they introduced a more rational approach based on the understanding of basic biochemical and physiological processes'.[23] Yet the history of rational drug design for antibiotics in particular has been humbling,[24] and no Nobel Prizes would ensue for antimicrobial therapeutics until the 2015 award (described below) to William Campbell, Satoshi Ōmura, and Tu Youyou, for drugs – avermectin, ivermectin, and artemisinin – initially discovered and even introduced well before 1988. Indeed, the discovery of artemisinin was explicitly framed as a nod to the insights of *ancient* Chinese medicine in many quarters.

Today, one could argue that there is no single paradigm or exemplar for antimicrobial drug discovery, as we find immunotherapeutics tasked alongside chemotherapy, antibiotics, and nucleoside analogs – as well as non-awarded remnants from the past like bacteriophage therapy and probiotics – in a broadening approach to infectious diseases, especially in the context of ever-growing concern over antimicrobial resistance. History has been both inspiring and sobering, tempering notions of the eradication of infectious diseases and encouraging a more humble, if creative and heterogeneous, approach to confronting infectious diseases.

Enduring Themes and Tensions

Yet despite such heterogeneity, there have been several key themes running throughout this history, and especially through the announcement of such prizes and therapeutics to the world. One theme, which is part of a more general discussion, has been the tension between the lone scientist versus the larger research group in the apportioning of credit; and antimicrobial therapeutic history has witnessed debates over proper credit ranging from von Behring versus Kitasato Shibasaburō in 1901, through Waksman versus Albert Schatz in 1952, to Youyou Tu versus her larger team in 2015.

Such tensions are perhaps exacerbated in the realm of therapeutics, which necessitates both laboratory discovery and clinical demonstration of efficacy.

---

23   Nobel Media AB 2014b.
24   Silver 2011; Lewis 2013.

And a focus on the lab and away from the social context in which diseases originate and are confronted, may well have been buttressed by the very metaphors used recurrently to describe such bacterial 'conquest': namely, military metaphors and especially the notion of the magic bullet. Such metaphors had already achieved prominence in bacteriology by the time the award was first presented,[25] but the Prize announcements certainly perpetuated their usage throughout the twentieth century. Count Mörner already noted in von Behring's presentation speech that von Behring's bacterial 'foe was obliged to drop his mask and make known his battle tactics', which von Behring countered with 'a reliable weapon against a developing disease'.[26] Behring himself, who had clashed with Rudolf Virchow by emphasizing an ontological view of disease (and therapeutic) specificity over Virchow's more contextualized nosology,[27] laid the groundwork for the magic bullet concept of eradicating the offending organism while sparing the host (and perhaps ignoring host factors), stating that 'because it does not influence the substrata of the diseased manifestations, the cells and organs, but only the *cause* of the disease, I call it aetiological therapy'.[28] And while von Behring would explicitly point to a time when scientific progress would remove 'the need of talking in parables', or metaphors, Ehrlich would coin the very term 'magic bullet' five years later to refer to the specificity of serotherapy and hoped-for chemotherapy.[29] By the time of Waksman's post-World War II award, Harald Cramér reported at the celebratory banquet that Waksman had 'discovered a new and powerful weapon in the deadly battle against one of the oldest foes of mankind. ...This battle is as old as medical science and we now have a definite impression that at last the enemy is beginning to yield'.[30] And Waksman himself, in his banquet speech, concluded:

I can do no better, in closing my remarks, than to quote from the words of the Founder [Alfred Nobel]: 'The advance in scientific research and its ever widening sphere stirs the hope in us that the microbes, those of the

---

25   Gradmann 2000.
26   Nobel Media AB 2014d.
27   Linton 2005.
28   Nobel Media AB 2014a; For the larger history in which this tension was embedded, see Carter 2003.
29   Paul De Kruif would inspire generations of would-be scientists with his 1926 classic, *Microbe Hunters*; and its concluding chapter on 'Paul Ehrlich: The Magic Bullet', would serve as the basis for the 1940 film, *Dr. Ehrlich's Magic Bullet*, starring Edward G. Robinson in the title role. See De Kruif 1926.
30   Nobel Media AB 2014e.

soul as well as of the body, will gradually disappear, and that the only war humanity will wage in the future will be one against these microbes'.[31]

Beyond such ballistic and military metaphors, the Nobel Prize for antimicrobial therapeutics has long drawn explicit attention to fundamental, rather than applied, aspects of antimicrobials, even if the clinical utility of such antimicrobials has always been an important consideration.[32] This tension was enunciated in the very first presentation speech to von Behring, when Count Mörner began by describing Alfred Nobel's hopes:

> The interest in medical science which was expressed in Alfred Nobel's will must have sprung from two roots. His heart was warmly inclined towards everything which could be of use and benefit to humanity. ... Closely connected with this, but also, one might say, as an independent feeling, was his love for scientific research.[33]

And for many years, the Nobel committees clearly prioritized the latter aspect – the novelty of fundamental research – over the delivery of the fruits of such research to those who need them the most.

Penicillin itself was presented as 'a splendid example of different scientific methods cooperating for a great common purpose. Once again it has shown us the fundamental importance of basic research. The starting-point was a purely academic investigation'.[34] The initial clinical investigators of streptomycin, Corwin Hinshaw and William Feldman, were nominated alongside Waksman for the 1947 award (admittedly by fellow Mayo clinicians), but only Waksman was awarded. In the Nobel Prize discussion of trimethoprim-sulfamethoxazole at the height of the AIDS epidemic in 1988, whereas the ingenious discovery of the inhibition of sequential steps in bacterial folate metabolism was emphasized, the drug's clinical utility appeared as a literal afterthought, when in the penultimate sentence of the presentation it was mentioned that 'it can be added that trimethoprim-sulfa is used in the treatment of Pneumocystis carinii, a relatively common complication to AIDS'.[35]

Yet such tension between basic and applied medical science was perhaps most famously exemplified in awards that were *not* given – to Jonas Salk and

---

31   Nobel Media AB 2014e.
32   Luttenberger 1996.
33   Nobel Media AB 2014d.
34   Nobel Media AB 2014c.
35   Nobel Media AB 2014b.

Albert Sabin for the introduction of the polio vaccine, and to Frank Fenner and others for the eradication of smallpox. As Erling Norrby and Stanley Prusiner have documented, while John Enders, Frederick Robbins, and Thomas Weller received the 1954 award for the growth of viruses in tissue culture, Salk and Sabin's accomplishments were considered more derivative, even if of immeasurable public health benefit.[36] When Frank Fenner, who had headed the World Health Organization team that had announced the eradication of smallpox, died in 2010, Nobelist Peter Doherty stated not that Fenner should have won the Nobel Prize in Physiology or Medicine, but rather that 'Fenner should have received the Nobel Peace Prize for his work eradicating smallpox `because they sometimes give the peace prize for enormous practical achievements'.[37]

A Shift?

But something seemingly shifted in 2015. At one level, over the past few decades, historians and scientists alike have drawn attention to the limitations – and even dangers – of the magic bullet metaphor and its allies. Allan Brandt, in his 1985 study, *No Magic Bullet* (explicitly concerned with syphilis, but published just as HIV had emerged on the global stage), drew attention to the social embeddedness of infectious diseases and the conditions that shaped and often frustrated the application of such wonder drugs as salvarsan and penicillin.[38] At another level, Joshua Lederberg, by the turn of the twenty-first century, turned our collective attention regarding microbes back upon and within us, challenging the Manichean view of 'We good; they evil' itself, and promoting the growing study of the 'microbiome' (a term coined by Lederberg the following year, in 2001) and the complicated relationships we maintain with such organisms.[39] Notions of magic bullets gave way to ecological considerations of the impacts (intended and unintended) of antimicrobials on their hosts' florae; and it is perhaps no accident that the 2015 Prize announcement was devoid of explicit ballistic or military metaphors.

But the 2015 Prize witnessed a still more profound shift, namely, towards the *global* application of remedies to help the world's most vulnerable individuals. Certainly, as Jeremy Greene has recently described, the 1960s and 1970s had already seen increasing attention devoted to the inequitable distribution of

---

36   Norrby and Prusiner 2007.
37   Maugh 2010.
38   Brandt 1985.
39   Lederberg 2000; Lederberg 2001.

life-saving remedies across the globe.[40] But such attention was not sustained, and only in the past two decades have we witnessed enduring attention to such global inequities, exemplified by the provision of antiretrovirals for treatment of HIV from the late 1990s onward, and by the formation of such programs as the Global Fund to Fight AIDS, Malaria, and Tuberculosis, as well as the President's Emergency Plan for AIDS Relief (PEPFAR). International health had become global health, involving such institutions as the WHO and the World Bank, federal governments, and innumerable non-governmental organizations (NGO's), and framed in some quarters as a moral necessity on behalf of the world's poorest individuals, in others as a pragmatic acknowledgment of the increasingly interconnected world of people and their infections, and in still others as a strategic component of foreign policy itself.[41]

Following and likely perpetuating this attention, the 2015 Prize was awarded to William Campbell and Satoshi Ōmura for the discoveries of avermectin and ivermectin – effective against river blindness and lymphatic filariasis – and to Youyou Tu for the discovery of artemisinin, effective against malaria. Simon Croft and Steven Ward, in their post-Prize account of the award in *Science Translational Medicine*, reminded their audiences that the mechanism of artemisinin wasn't even known yet, while in the Karolinska Institute's 'Scientific Background' piece to the Prize it was noted that 'the mode of Ivermectin is not known in detail'.[42] So something else was at stake, and in the official announcement of the award, it was the *global health* needs seemingly addressed by the drugs, rather than any novel biological mechanism per se, that was emphasized. The Nobel Prize press release began: 'Diseases caused by parasites have plagued humankind for millennia and constitute a major global health problem. In particular, parasitic diseases affect the world's poorest populations and represent a huge barrier to improving human health and wellbeing'.[43] The very 'Scientific Background' piece by the Nobel Assembly at the Karolinska Institute continued in this vein. In discussing Avermectin, its authors noted:

> More than one billion people world-wide are infected with one or more species of intestinal nematodes. These diseases hamper economic growth and result in a major public health burden which disproportionately

---

40   Greene 2016.
41   Brown, Cueto, Fee 2006; Packard 2016.
42   Croft and Ward 2015; Andersson, Forssberg, Zierath 2015.
43   Nobel Media AB 2014g.

affects the poor and are considered diseases of neglected communities and neglected people.[44]

Reflecting two decades of attention to HIV, malaria, and TB, and a social medicine ethos absent from over a century of Nobel announcements regarding antimicrobials, the authors concluded:

> The global impact of Avermectin and Artemisinin treatment goes far beyond reducing the disease burden of individual people. These parasitic diseases place an enormous disease burden that disproportionately affects the poor and vulnerable. In particular, they place a life-long burden on the inflicted individual by depriving them of the opportunity to gain an education and acquisition of the necessary skill sets to support themselves and their families, further oppressing them and committing them to a life of poverty. Thus, these diseases not only lead to chronic illness, they are also associated with physical and mental disabilities that hamper an individual's overall health, wellbeing and economic livelihood. ...The discoveries of [the] 2015 Nobel Laureates represents a paradigm shift in medicine, which has not only provided a revolutionary therapy for patients suffering from devastating parasitic diseases, but it has also promoted wellbeing and prosperity of both individuals and society. The global impact of their discoveries and the benefit to mankind is immeasurable.[45]

Indeed, Croft and Ward, writing from schools of tropical medicine and concerned with treatment of neglected tropical diseases, hoped that the awarding of the 2015 Prize would 'act to reinvigorate support for research and development efforts across the entire tropical disease portfolio', reasoning that

> in an era in which future Nobel Prize-winning initiatives are undoubtedly underway focusing on strategies that can relegate these infections to the history books ... [the efforts of the 2015 prize-winners] ... will be cited as the driving exemplars of what could be achieved with the appropriate tools **delivered** to those that need them (emphasis added).[46]

---

44   Andersson, Forssberg, Zierath 2015.
45   Ibid.
46   Croft and Ward 2015.

On the one hand, such statements, along with the drawing of attention to global health needs in the first place, would seem at least to point to the need for rigorously evaluated delivery science as a critical component of global health. As Jim Kim, Paul Farmer, and Michael Porter have recently stated:

> The gritty business of actually delivering health care in developing countries has not attracted much academic interest, even though improving capacity to deliver care in these settings will save lives, leverage substantial and growing philanthropic support of global health, and increase returns on existing and new investments in both discovery and development of new resources.[47]

Neglected communities and neglected people necessitated that renewed attention be given to the settings in which diseases originated and in which care was to be delivered, along with rigorous evaluation of the means and value of delivering care to such individuals. It should be noted, along these lines, that the treatment of both river blindness with ivermectin, and malaria with artemisinin (in combination with other anti-malarials), have been achieved through the use of community health workers.[48]

On the other hand, while neither ivermectin nor artemisinin may have been explicitly described as a 'magic bullet' per se, they were indeed framed as such in all but name in the official Nobel Prize announcements described above. Randall Packard, in his studies of the history of malaria and of global health more broadly, has drawn attention to the longstanding tension between those focused on discrete biomedical technological solutions to such particular diseases as smallpox, malaria, and HIV, and those focused on the strengthening of local health systems (including staff and facilities) that can underpin the diagnosis and treatment of present and future plagues alike. Over most of the twentieth century, the former approach has served as the focus of most global health efforts, from the campaign to eliminate smallpox to PEPFAR, and from river blindness to malaria.[49] The official discourse surrounding the 2015 Nobel Prize in Physiology or Medicine would seem, at least explicitly, to echo this ethos.

It is difficult to tease out the degree to which the awarding of, and announcements regarding, the Nobel Prize in Physiology or Medicine over the past 118 years have reflected or driven our ideals of, and priorities concerning,

---

47   Kim, Farmer, Porter 2013.
48   Meredith, Cross, Amazigo 2012; Kamal-Yanni, Potet, Saunders 2012.
49   Packard 2007; Packard 2016.

antimicrobial therapy, and especially our historical lack of attention to delivery science and the structures in which care is embedded. It seems likely that it has done both, and that given the Nobel Prize's prominence, it has the capacity to continue to draw attention to magic bullets and technological solutions, as well as to the enduring delivery aspects of antimicrobials around the world. As this volume illustrates, the awarding of the Nobel Prizes in Physiology or Medicine has been a fluid, evolving process, and the distinction between 'medicine' and broader measures to ensure global health and prosperity has become ever murkier. Whether the arbiters of the Nobel Prize in Physiology or Medicine will go so far one day as to award a Prize for delivery science remains to be seen.

Bibliography

Andersson, J.; Forssberg, H.; Zierath, J.R. 2015. 'Scientific Background: Avermectin and Artemisinin: Revolutionary Therapies against Parasitic Diseases'. https://www.nobelprize. org/nobel_prizes/medicine/laureates/2015/advanced-medicineprize2015.pdf (accessed February 21, 2019).

Behforouz, H.L.; Farmer, P.E.; Mukherjee, J.S. 2004. 'From Directly Observed Therapy to Accompagnateurs: Enhancing AIDS Treatment Outcomes in Haiti and in Boston'. *Clinical Infectious Diseases* 38: S429–S436.

Brandt, A.M. 1985. *No Magic Bullet. A Social History of Venereal Disease in the United States since 1880.* New York: Oxford University Press.

Brown, T.M.; Cueto, M.; Fee, E. 2006. 'The World Health Organization and the Transition from 'International' to 'Global' Health'. *American Journal of Public Health* 96: 62–72.

Bud, R. 2007. *Penicillin: Triumph and Tragedy.* New York: Oxford University Press.

Burnet, F.M. 1962. *Natural History of Infectious Disease (Third Edition).* Cambridge: Cambridge University Press.

Carter, C.K. 2003. 'The Rise of Causal Concepts of Disease: Case Histories'. *Social History of Medicine* 16(3): 529–530.

Croft S.L. and Ward, S. 2015. 'The Nobel Prize in Medicine 2015: Two Drugs that Changed Global Health'. *Science Translational Medicine* 7: 316ed14.

Daemmrich, A. 2009. 'Synthesis by Microbes or Chemists? Pharmaceutical Research and Manufacturing in the Antibiotic Era'. *History and Technology* 25: 237–256.

Ehrlich, P. 1906 [1960]. 'Address Delivered at the Dedication of the Georg-Speyer-Haus'. In *The Collected Papers of Paul Ehrlich, Volume III*, edited by F. Himmelweit, 53–63. New York: Pergammon Press.

Farmer, P. 2013. 'Accompaniment as Public Policy'. In *To Repair the World: Paul Farmer Speaks to the Next Generation*, edited by J. Weigel, 233–247. Berkeley: University of California Press.

Fleming, A. 1945. 'Penicillin', Nobel Prize Lecture, December 11. http://www.nobelprize
.org/uploads/2018/06/fleming-lecture.pdf (accessed February 21, 2019).

Gradmann, C. 2000. 'Invisible Enemies: Bacteriology and the Language of Politics in
Imperial Germany'. *Science in Context* 13: 9–30.

Gray, J.D. and Fulton, M.C. 1938. 'The Mortality and Treatment of Lobar Pneumonia'.
Journal of the Medical Association of Georgia 27: 419–420.

Greene, J.A. 2016. 'Pharmaceutical Geographies: Mapping the Boundaries of the
Therapeutic Revolution'. In *Therapeutic Revolutions: Pharmaceuticals and Social
Change in the Twentieth Century*, edited by J.A. Greene, F. Condrau and E.S. Watkins,
150–185. Chicago: University of Chicago Press.

Grundmann, E. 2004. *Gerhard Domagk: The First Man to Triumph over Infectious
Diseases*. Münster: LIT.

Hróbjartsson, A.; Gøtzsche, P.C.; Gludd, C. 1998. 'The Controlled Clinical Trial Turns
100 Years: Fibiger's Trial of Serum Treatment of Diphtheria'. *British Medical Journal*
317: 1243–1245.

Kamal-Yanni, M.M.; Potet, J.; Saunders, P.M. 2012. 'Scaling-up Malaria Treatment: A Review of the Performance of Different Providers'. *Malaria Journal* 11: 414.

Kim, J.Y.; Farmer, P.; Porter, M.E. 2013. 'Redefining Global Health-Care Delivery'. *Lancet*
382: 1060–1069.

De Kruif, P. 1926. *Microbe Hunters*. New York: Harcourt, Brace, and Company.

Lederberg, J. 2000. 'Infectious History'. *Science* 288: 287–293.

Lederberg, J. 2001. 'Beyond the Genome'. *Brooklyn Law Review* 67: 7–12.

Lesch, J.E. 2007. *The First Miracle Drugs: How the Sulfa Drugs Transformed Medicine*.
New York: Oxford University Press.

Lewis, K. 2013. 'Platforms for Antibiotic Discovery'. *Nature Reviews Drug Discovery* 12:
371–387.

Linton, D.S. 2005. *Emil Von Behring: Infectious Disease, Immunology, Serum Therapy*.
Philadelphia: American Philosophical Society.

Lown, B. 2008. *Prescription for Survival: A Doctor's Journey to End Nuclear Madness*. San
Francisco: Berrett-Koehler Publishers.

Luttenberger, F. 1996. 'Excellence and Chance: The Nobel Prize Case of E. von Behring
and É. Roux'. *History and Philosophy of the Life Sciences* 18: 225–238.

Maugh, T.H. 2010. 'Frank Fenner dies at 95; Microbiologist Led the Eradication of
Smallpox'. *Los Angeles Times*, 28 November.

Meredith, S.E.; Cross, C.; Amazigo, U.V. 2012. 'Empowering Communities in Combating
River Blindness: Case Studies from Cameroon, Mali, Nigeria, and Uganda'. *Health
Research Policy and Systems* 10: 16.

Mitnick, C.D.; Shin, S.S.; Seung, K.J. et al. 2008. 'Comprehensive Treatment of Extensively
Drug-Resistant Tuberculosis'. *New England Journal of Medicine* 359: 563–574.

Nobel Media AB. 2014a. 'Emil von Behring – Nobel Lecture: Serum Therapy in Therapeutics and Medical Science'. http://www.nobelprize.org/nobel_prizes/medicine/laureates/1901/behring-lecture.html (accessed February 21, 2019).

Nobel Media AB. 2014b. 'Physiology or Medicine 1988 – Press Release'. http://www.nobelprize.org/nobel_prizes/medicine/laureates/1988/press.html (accessed February 21, 2019).

Nobel Media AB. 2014c. 'Physiology or Medicine 1945 – Presentation Speech'. http://www.nobelprize.org/nobel_prizes/medicine/laureates/1945/press.html (accessed February 21, 2019).

Nobel Media AB. 2014d. 'The Nobel Prize in Physiology or Medicine 1901 – Presentation Speech'. http://www.nobelprize.org/nobel_prizes/medicine/laureates/1901/press.html (accessed February 21, 2019).

Nobel Media AB. 2014e. 'Selman A. Waksman – Banquet Speech'. http://www.nobelprize.org/nobel_prizes/medicine/laureates/1952/waksman-speech.html (accessed February 21, 2019).

Nobel Media AB. 2014f. 'Physiology or Medicine 1939 – Presentation Speech'. http://www.nobelprize.org/nobel_prizes/medicine/laureates/1939/press.html (accessed February 21, 2019).

Nobel Media AB. 2014g. 'The 2015 Nobel Prize in Physiology or Medicine – Press Release'. http://www.nobelprize.org/nobel_prizes/medicine/laureates/2015/press.html (accessed February 21, 2019).

Norrby, E. and Prusiner, S.B. 2007. 'Polio and Nobel Prizes: Looking Back 50 Years'. *Annals of Neurology* 61: 385–395.

Packard, R.M. 2007. *The Making of a Tropical Disease: A Short History of Malaria*. Baltimore: Johns Hopkins University Press.

Packard, R.M. 2016. *A History of Global Health: Interventions into the Lives of Other Peoples*. Baltimore: Johns Hopkins University Press.

Podolsky, S.H. 2006. *Pneumonia before Antibiotics: Therapeutic Evolution and Evaluation in Twentieth-Century America*. Baltimore: Johns Hopkins University Press.

Podolsky, S.H. 2015. *The Antibiotic Era: Reform, Resistance, and the Pursuit of a Rational Therapeutics*. Baltimore: Johns Hopkins University Press.

Podolsky, S.H. and Kveim Lie, A. 2016. 'Futures and their Uses: Antibiotics and Therapeutic Revolutions'. In *Therapeutic Revolutions: Pharmaceuticals and Social Change in the Twentieth Century*, edited by J.A. Greene, F. Condrau and E.S. Watkins, 18–42. Chicago: University of Chicago Press.

Potts, W.H. 1937. 'Serum Therapy in Lobar Pneumonia'. *Texas State Journal of Medicine* 33: 418–422.

Pringle, P. 2012. *Experiment Eleven: Dark Secrets Behind the Discovery of a Wonder Drug*. New York: Walker and Company.

Salomon-Bayet, C. 1982. 'Bacteriology and Nobel Prize Selections, 1901–1920'. In *Science, Technology, and Society in the Time of Alfred Nobel*, edited by C.G. Bernhard, E. Crawford, P. Sörbom, 377–400. Oxford: Pergamon Press.

Sherwood Taylor, F. 1942. *The Conquest of Bacteria: From Salvarsan to Sulphapyridine.* New York: Philosophical Library and Alliance Book Corporation.

Shin, S.S.; Furin, J.; Bayona, J. et al. 2004. 'Community-based Treatment of Multidrug-resistant Tuberculosis in Lima, Peru: 7 years of Experience'. *Social Sciences & Medicine* 59: 1529–1539.

Silver, L.L. 2011. 'Challenges of Antibacterial Discovery'. *Clinical Microbiology Reviews* 24: 71–109.

Spellberg, B. 2008. 'Dr. William H. Stewart: Mistaken or Maligned?' *Clinical Infectious Diseases* 47: 294.

Waksman, S.A. 1973. 'History of the Word 'Antibiotic''. *Journal of the History of Medicine* 28: 284–286.

CHAPTER 5

Discovery or Reputation? Jacques Loeb and the Role of Nomination Networks

Heiner Fangerau, Thorsten Halling and Nils Hansson

A 2015 contribution to the Journal of the American Medical Association (JAMA) raised the question of why American Nobel Laureates outnumber those of any other nativity.[1] Times are changing. About 100 years ago, when the Prize was quite new, the same journal asked why only European scientists were acknowledged.[2] At that time, U.S. medical journals praised the Nobel Prize as 'the ideal method of encouraging the best scientific research'[3] and used it as a yardstick for other medical honours. Commentators repeatedly bemoaned that American research 'of fundamental importance'[4] had been disregarded. Whether for the prize money (corresponding to about one million USD) or the international competition in science and medicine, the Prize was perceived as a coveted trophy right from its inception.[5]

It is not as if Americans did not nominate domestic candidates. In fact, JAMA even published calls to name Walter Reed and James Carrol for their investigations into yellow fever.[6] However, another American candidate would eventually come to play a larger role in the nomination cycle. The physiologist Jacques Loeb (1859–1924) was, according to the Nomination Database of the Nobel Committee for Physiology or Medicine, nominated 78 times between 1901 and his death,[7] which makes him one of the most nominated scholars in the first half of the 20th century.[8] Nevertheless, Loeb was, as Robert Merton phrased it in his classical paper on the Matthew effect, an occupant of the '41st chair'.[9]

---

1   Naylor and Bell 2015.
2   Anon 1905.
3   Anon 1903.
4   Anon 1905.
5   Halling, Fangerau, Hansson 2018.
6   Anon 1904.
7   Fangerau 2010, 183.
8   17 additional nominations arrived too late to be included in the Nobel committee's decisions.
9   Merton used the example of the French Academy of Science and their early decision that 'only a cohort of 40 could qualify as members and so emerge as immortals' in order to describe the 'artifact of having a fixed number of places available at the summit of recognition' (Merton 1968).

In 1951, the former Secretary of the Nobel Committee, pharmacologist Göran Liljestrand, gave a short explanation as to why Loeb (according to his opinion) never made it. He wrote that 'the examiners [...] remained unconvinced as to [...] [the] scope and general significance' of his work. On the other hand, he stressed that 'between 1901 and 1924, Loeb was proposed for a Nobel Prize by about a hundred sponsors in ten different countries'.[10]

One should bear in mind that the sheer number of Nobel Prize nominations gives a first hint of a researcher's worldwide reputation and recognition. Furthermore, a substantial amount of nominations might even increase the chances to be awarded. The early American Nobel complaints in JAMA, Merton's Matthew effect and Liljestrand's remark on the number of nominees reflect a common idea about why certain scientists receive the Prize for Physiology or Medicine and others do not: the final selection depends on networks of nominees. The underlying hypothesis is that because science is not just a cognitive activity but also a social endeavour, the effects of social processes in prize politics need to be examined to understand why research is considered prize-worthy or why the contribution of a scientist remains disputed.

In our chapter, we will address this hypothesis using the example of Jacques Loeb and his nominations. We will ask who nominated him and for what reason and describe some of the links that connected the nominators with Loeb. Additionally, we will examine how the Nobel committee's referees evaluated the nominations. A Loeb case study is particularly suitable for such an investigation not only because of the rich archival files on him but first and foremost because it highlights disciplinary conflicts (struggles in the grey areas between morphology, chemistry, biology and experimental physiology) and scientific priority disputes in the first two decades of the 20th century.[11] From a historical perspective, it is unusual for a candidate to be awarded after only a few nominations. Normally, the Nobel committee watched their front-runners for several years before making a decision (see the chapter by Fabio De Sio et al. on Nobel laureate John C. Eccles in this volume). During the years in which Loeb had been nominated, some requirements were repeatedly stressed in evaluative reports following a first selection of him as a potential candidate (see Introduction). It should be a fresh discovery, and it should have potential to open up new scientific avenues of research. It was also crucial that the discovery in question be verified by the scientific community and that issues of priority were settled.

---

10   Liljestrand 1962, 242.
11   On Loeb, his science and struggles see Pauly 1987; Rasmussen and Tilman 1998; Fangerau 2010.

We will analyse whether the nominators addressed these points and we will reconstruct Loeb's nomination network. Loeb was a disputatious character who fought for his scientific convictions in a polemical manner. At the same time, he had powerful supporters and friends. An analysis of his Nobel nominations will offer a better understanding for how reputable his research really was among medical scientists. With the help of this case, we come to some conclusions regarding the value of nomination networks for understanding the intellectual and social organisation or the reputational system of the Nobel Prize.[12]

Sources

The starting point of our analysis is the material on Loeb in the Archive of the Nobel Committee for Physiology or Medicine, which includes nomination dossiers as well as four reports by members of the Nobel Committee written in 1906, 1909 and two in 1917. Most of the nominations are written in English or German, and all evaluations in Swedish. The original documents are not accessible – only copies which have been transcribed by Swedish staff of the Nobel Committee and bound together in yearbooks. Therefore, we cannot investigate marginalia or corrections. Nevertheless, we get as close as possible to the decisions of the Nobel Committee.

The Swedish historian Franz Luttenberger was one of the first scholars to explore the Nobel Archive for Physiology or Medicine.[13] He focused on files concerning Svante Arrhenius, Paul Ehrlich, Emil von Behring and Émile Roux. His work is of particular interest for this study since the formal statutes in the Nobel Committee of the early 20th century concern Loeb as well: the International Nominating System, the Nobel Committee and evaluative reports. At the beginning of the century every year, all professors of medicine in Scandinavia were invited to nominate a scholar for the Nobel Prize in Physiology or Medicine. This right was also enjoyed by the Faculty members of the Karolinska Institute, and a few leading universities and scientific associations. The job of the Nobel Committee consisted of agreeing on one candidate mentioned in the nominations, whom they proposed to the Faculty. As a basis, the committee first agreed on a shortlist with usually five to fifteen candidates. In order for the Nobel Committee to get a nuanced view of Loeb's work, experts discussed the statements of the nominators and the strengths and weakness of his methods. However, Loeb's research was also brought up in Nobel Committee reports

---

12   Whitley 2000, 11.
13   Luttenberger 1996.

about other scholars, such as the one on surgeon Alexis Carrel in 1912.[14] In the discussion over Carrel's experiments with tissue culture, competitors like Loeb and Ross Granville Harrison (1870–1959) played a part. These reports offer a mediated perspective on how Loeb's achievements were interpreted during these years.

Jacques Loeb and the Nobel Prize

Jacques Loeb was born in Germany and educated as a physiologist.[15] After completing his studies in medicine, he worked as an assistant of Nathan Zuntz in Berlin (1885), Adolf Fick in Würzburg (1886–1888) and Friedrich Goltz in Straßburg (1888–1891). In 1891, he emigrated to the United States. In letters to Ernst Mach and other colleagues and friends, he attributed his emigration to the rigid hierarchical structures of German universities and the anti-Semitism in German academia which made it difficult for him to find a permanent appointment.[16] In the United States, he held positions at Bryn Mawr, Chicago (1882), Berkeley (1902) and finally at the Rockefeller Institute for Medical Research (1910), which offered a unique and innovative research atmosphere.[17] During his scientific life, Loeb developed his own research programme of 'general physiology' directed at investigating life phenomena by reducing them to the laws of physics and chemistry. Furthermore, he intended to apply these laws in order to synthesise living matter – 'that is, to form new combinations from the elements of living nature, just as the physicist and chemist form new combinations from the elements of non-living nature'.[18] The construction of life meant for him fully understanding its underlying processes. Based on a quantitative, experimental approach to biology,[19] he followed an ideal that Philip Pauly referred to as Loeb's 'engineering standpoint'.[20]

Loeb gained world-wide recognition for his research on tropisms (induced conduct) in the animal kingdom and for studies on directed regeneration and heteromorphosis during the 1880s and 1890s, but he became a real

---

14   Yearbook 1912 (Nobel Archive).
15   For the following short biography see Fangerau and Müller 2005; Fangerau 2009.
16   Pauly 1987, chap. 2, 55ff.
17   Hollingsworth 2004.
18   Loeb 1912d, 109.
19   Loeb 1912b; Loeb 1912c, 3–4.
20   Pauly 1987, 8.

science celebrity[21] or a 'visible scientist'[22] after having succeeded in inducing development in sea urchin eggs without sperm in 1899. He called this process artificial parthenogenesis.[23] Although Loeb did research on such different fields as brain physiology, regeneration, antagonistic salt actions, duration of life, proteins and colloidal behaviour, his work on artificial parthenogenesis had the most sustainable legacy. As Liljestrand recalls, most of the nominators for the Nobel Prize 'particularly stressed' these works.[24] Newspapers and magazines like the New York Times, the Chicago Tribune and the Cosmopolitan reported on him and his 'chemical creation of life'.[25] The Viennese physicist Ludwig Boltzmann joked in his 1905 travelling reports from the United States of America on how he embarrassed young women with Loeb's findings over dinner.[26] Other scientists, like Wilhelm Roux, again commented carefully on the exaggerated press reports.[27]

After the turn of the century, Jacques Loeb was a well-known and highly reputed representative of physiology. Scientists from all over the world visited his laboratories while he was at Berkeley (among them eminent scientists from various disciplines, like Hugo de Vries, Ludwig Boltzmann, Ernest Rutherford and Nathan Zuntz). Loeb was under consideration by colleagues for chairs in Halle, Berlin and Budapest before he took a prestigious position at the Rockefeller Institute for Medical Research (RIMR) in 1910. In 1909 he received honorary doctorates from Cambridge, Geneva and Leipzig. By 1914 he had become an honorary member in numerous international scientific societies. He was in correspondence with laureates like Svante Arrhenius (Nobel Prize in Chemistry in 1903), Paul Ehrlich (Nobel Prize in Physiology or Medicine 1908), and, until the beginning of the First World War, a friend of Wilhelm Ostwald (Nobel Prize in Chemistry 1909), whose son Wolfgang worked in Loeb's laboratory between 1904 and 1906.[28] All in all, due to his artificial parthenogenesis experiment, Loeb had reached a popularity peak when the first Nobel Prize was to be announced in December 1901. Additionally, he was to increase his scientific symbolic capital during the next years. The question persists: why didn't the nominations between 1901 and 1924 bear fruit?

---

21   Pauly 1987, 100.
22   Turney 1995, 156; Bucchi 2015.
23   Loeb 1899.
24   Liljestrand 1962, 242.
25   Turney 1995, 156.
26   Fangerau 2010, 213.
27   Turney 1995, 159.
28   Pauly 1987, 113; Fangerau 2010, 39.

Nominations

Alfred Nobel had stipulated that the Prize should reflect research that had been presented during the 'preceding year', and the fortunate timing of Loeb's publication on artificial parthenogenesis might be a factor as to why Loeb was the only US-based nominee for the first Nobel Prize in Physiology or Medicine. He was put forward by two sponsors, the Johns Hopkins embryologist and anatomist Franklin P. Mall and the Harvard psychologist Hugo Münsterberg. Mall directly referred to Loeb's *discovery of artificial parthenogenesis*. Münsterberg declared in a detailed nomination that Loeb was the only person who had deserved the Prize because his works were the only ones that contributed visionary new perspectives to physiology. However, Münsterberg did not concentrate on artificial parthenogenesis alone, but delivered a whole bibliography, which he categorised in works related to the chemical effects of electricity, to the effects of ions, to oxidation in the cell, to development and to the central nervous system. He compared Loeb's contributions to those of Hermann von Helmholtz, Robert Koch, Wilhelm Wundt, Charles Richet and Rudolf Virchow, but stressed that Loeb's works were much more recent and that he would consider it an awkward solution if one of the other famous gentlemen were to get the Prize for work which belongs to the past. Additionally, Münsterberg weaved an international aspect into his nomination. Referring to Loeb's emigration from Germany, which he in part explained by referring to controversies Loeb had had within the German scientific community, he argued that awarding Loeb would show younger scholars that it might be worthwhile to rise against the mainstream of research and the narrowmindedness of regional scientific cliques. When Loeb, under pressure, had to leave Germany, this narrow-minded republic of scholars ('kleinliche Gelehrtenrepublik') had scored a victory. Now the Nobel committee had the chance of proving that it could serve as a scientific clearing board. Awarding Loeb would be a statement that scientific ideas were more powerful than a German clique. Consequently, he wrote, a Prize for Loeb would do science a service, even more so since a German prize awarded to Loeb by the Senckenberg Institute in Frankfurt could not be accepted by him because this could only be accepted by German citizens. Besides arguments based on Loeb's works, he indirectly put forward the argument of internationalism in science as a criterion for his nomination.

The Nobel committee did not follow Münsterberg's advice, perhaps due to the strong emphasis on European scientists in the other nominations. A review of the nomination letters for 1901 reveals that the Prize was not international in practice. For example, eleven scholars from Germany, six from Austria and three from Sweden were proposed. In the end, the German physiologist Emil von Behring was chosen for his work on serum therapy and its application against diphtheria.[29]

Loeb's sponsors did not surrender. Over the following two decades, further nominations were sent to Stockholm, primarily by American scientists. John Auer argued in 1913 that Loeb had unravelled 'the mechanisms of Life', and Loeb's director at the RIMR Simon Flexner proposed him eight times between 1913 and 1922. His colleagues at the RIMR – Phoebus Levene, Samuel J. Meltzer and Alexis Carrel – also sent nomination letters to Stockholm. Close friends, former colleagues and relatives nominated him as well. Loeb received nominations, for example, in 1902 by the physiologist Justus Gaule from Zurich, who was married to the older sister of Loeb's wife, and in 1909 and 1912 by his former co-assistant in Friedrich Goltz's laboratory Alexander Koranyi, with whom he stayed in rather close contact during these years.[30] Another nominator who had been working with Loeb in Goltz's laboratory was Ernst Julius Richard Ewald, who nominated him twice.

According to the Nobel prize database, Loeb received 78 nominations from 54 scientists from eight countries over the following years.[31] The database lists nominators, nominees, the year of the nomination, the affiliation of nominee and nominator and a summarising account of the reason for the proposal. Surely, the database has its limitations in its reduction and some minor mistakes. Nevertheless, its value for a summary account is unquestioned. In addition to the database, we analysed most of the nominations in the Nobel Archives. According to the database, Loeb received 29 nominations from the USA, 13 from Germany, 11 from France and 11 from the Austrian-Hungarian Kingdom. A further 4 were from Italy, another 4 from Russia (including Estonia, Russia at that time), 3 from Belgium and 3 from Switzerland.

A further 17 nominations, however, are not listed in the database. They belong to the so-called *Group VII* in the nomination files of the Nobel Archives. These are nominations which reached the Nobel committee after the closing date for nominations on the 31st of January. Often these nominations were only a couple of days too late.[32] They are also kept in the Nomination files. The US-American chemist Julius Stieglitz in 1917 gave as a reason for the delayed transfer of reprints of Loeb's works that he needed consent from the British embassy. Giving this reason, he 'trust[ed] that this delay will not invalidate

---

29   Enke 2018.
30   Loeb for example seems to have been in close contact with Koranyi during a journey to Europe (correspondence Loeb to Emil Godlewski, jr. 20.07.1909 (Archives Jagiellonian Universiy Kraków, DIV 76); Wolfgang Ostwald to Loeb 24.08.1909 (Library of Congress (LC), Manuscript Division, Loeb Papers).
31   For the following figures and numbers see also Fangerau 2010, 183–189.
32   Halling, Hansson, Fangerau 2018, 80.

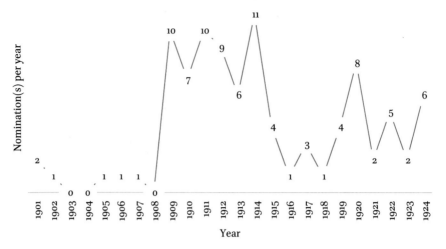

FIGURE 5.1   Nomination(s) for Loeb per year

Dr. Loeb's candidacy, especially in view of the extraordinary' war conditions.[33] Some other nominators explicitly referred to these excluded nominations, when they were asked again during the following years to submit a nomination. Alexis Carrel, for example, in a nomination from 1922 referred to a complete selection of reprints of Loeb's works, which he had sent in 1921 in a nomination, which ended up in Group VII. As the nominations were filed and nominators referred to them, Group VII nominations most probably found their way to the Nobel committee and were considered. Therefore, we included these 17 nominations and 4 additional nominators in the following analysis.[34]

Most of the nominations for Loeb were sent to Stockholm between 1909 and 1914. During the War, the number of nominations decreased substantially.[35] From 1915 to 1918, in general, fewer nominations for the Nobel Prize in Physiology or Medicine were submitted.[36] According to Liljestrand, this was due to the 'extreme confusion that prevailed throughout Europe'[37] as a consequence of the First World War. After the War, the number began to rise again (Figure 5.1).

Loeb received most of his nominations from the USA. Especially after the war, the US-share increased to over 50% (Figure 5.2).

---

33   Yearbook 1918 (Nobel Archive).
34   They were not included in a previous study (Fangerau 2010), which solely was based on the 78 official nominations which can also be found in the database.
35   See chap. 3 in this volume.
36   1910: 136 Nom.; 1911: 91; 1912: 108; 1913: 136; 1914: 151; 1915: 61; 1916: 64; 1917: 75; 1918: 104; 1919: 104; 1920: 125. No awards between 1915–1918.
37   Liljestrand 1962, 168.

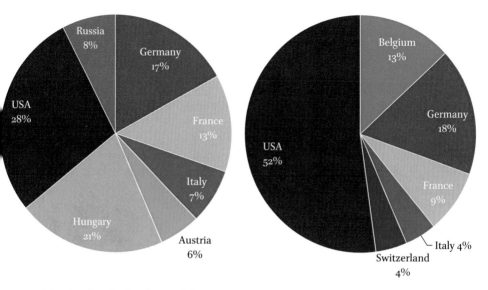

FIGURE 5.2   Nominations by countries

Most nominations for Loeb referred to his work on artificial parthenogenesis. In addition, his works on tropism and his works on colloidal behaviour are mentioned as prize-worthy (Table 5.1). Some simply state that no motivation is necessary, because his works were 'pathbreaking' (Julius Richard Ewald in 1914), everybody knew Loeb's work (Franz Hofmeister in 1915) or they nominated him for all the work he had done.

The length of the nominations varies substantially. Some, like Münsterberg's from 1901 or Ladislaus von Udranszky's from 1912 and 1913 (almost the same text in both years), are several pages long and include a long list of literature. Others are just one sentence, which is repeated over the years, if a nominator was asked for a nomination again. Phoebus Levene, for example, in 1914 just wrote: 'In reply to your letter of Sept 1913 I wish to nominate as candidate for the year 1914 Doctor Jacques Loeb for his work on artificial fertilisation. Very respectfully...'. He repeated this sentence twice, once in a nomination for 1919, and for the year 1920.[38]

Altogether, 58 colleagues proposed Loeb to the Nobel committee. Some were able to do so more than once (Table 5.2). Most often, Loeb was suggested as a single candidate, but not always. Albrecht Bethe (another of Goltz' assistants), for example, in his nomination from 1923 listed almost a dozen names,

---

38   Loeb himself also wrote only one sentence when he had the chance to give a nomination in 1914. He suggested very briefly his colleague from the RIMR Samuel J. Meltzer for his work on 'anaesthesia and insufflation', Yearbook 1914 (Nobel Archive).

TABLE 5.1   Reasons for nominating Loeb (sometimes more than one reason is given in the
             nomination. Therefore, in 95 nominations we found 147 reasons).

Reason	N	%	first year	last year
Artificial Parthenogenesis	54	37%	1901	1922
Tropism	14	10%	1909	1920
Chemistry of fertilisation	8	5%	1909	1923
Physical chemistry applied in physiology	8	5%	1910	1924
Colloid chemistry and proteins	8	5%	1921	1924
Physiological (experimental) Morphology/ Biology	7	5%	1901	1924
Developmental Physiology	5	3%	1901	1919
No motivation	5	3%	1909	1915
General physiology	5	3%	1911	1921
Effect of ions	5	3%	1912	1922
Biology	5	3%	1912	1922
Dynamics of living matter	4	3%	1909	1923
Heterogeneous hybridization	4	3%	1909	1918
Role of ions for nerve and muscle function	2	1%	1901	1910
Effects of electric stimulation	2	1%	1901	1913
Brain physiology	2	1%	1901	1919
Antagonistic action of salts	2	1%	1909	1913
All the work Loeb has done	2	1%	1912	1917
Role of salts in the preservation of life	2	1%	1913	1913
Oxidation in the cell	1	1%	1901	
Comparative physiology	1	1%	1905	
Effect of physical agents on organisms	1	1%	1919	

and Charles Richet nominated Loeb together with Maurice Arthus, (1921, 1922), Charles Sherrington (1921, 1922), Yves Delage (1915) and Hartog J. Hamburger (1921).

Loeb knew most of his nominators personally, either as former colleagues and friends (see Koranyi and Gaule above, Stieglitz in Chicago), as mentors (for example Nathan Zuntz) or as alumni at the Rockefeller Institute of Medical Research (for example Simon Flexner, Alexis Carell, Phoebus Levene, Samuel Meltzer, John Auer). Existing connections with Julius Richard Ewald, for example, were intensified just before Ewald's second nomination in 1914 when

TABLE 5.2   Loeb's nominators[a]

Number of nominations	Nominator	Discipline	first year	last year
8	Flexner, Simon	Bacteriology	1913	1922
6	Wassermann, August von	Serology	1909	1920
5	Levene, Phoebus A.	Physiological Chemistry	1914	1920
3	Carrel, Alexis	Surgery	1922	1924
3	Galeotti, Gino	General Pathology	1910	1920
3	Gaule, Justus	Physiology	1902	1915
3	Grosz, Emile de	Ophthalmiatrics	1909	1914
3	Mall, Franklin P.	Anatomy	1901	1910
3	Richet, Charles R.	Physiology	1915	1922
3	Tangl, Franz	Physiology	1907	1914
2	Bottazzi, Filippo	Experimental Physiology	1910	1914
2	Ewald, Julius Richard	Physiology	1910	1914
2	Koranyi, Alexander	Internal Medicine	1909	1912
2	Mesnil, Felix	Zoology	1909	1910
2	Stieglitz, Julius	Chemistry	1909	1918
2	Tandler, Julius M.	Anatomy	1912	1914
2	Udranszky, Ladislaus von	Physiology	1912	1913
1	Asher, Leon	Physiology	1920	
1	Auer, John	Physiology	1913	
1	Bataillon, Eugene	General Biology	1919	
1	Bethe, Albrecht	Physiology	1923	
1	Blumer, George	Clinical Medicine	1911	
1	Bluntschli, Hans	Anatomy	1923	
1	Brachet, Albert	Anatomy	1924	
1	Caullery, Maurice	General Biology	1912	
1	Dogiel, Alexandre S.	Histology	1911	
1	Dollinger, Julius	Dermatology	1913	
1	Flint, Joseph M.	Practical Surgery	1911	
1	Franqué, Otto von	Gynecology	1911	
1	Garten, Siegfried	Physiology	1911	
1	Gérard, Pol	Histology	1924	
1	Hertel, Ernst	Ophthalmiatrics	1914	
1	Hofmeister, Franz	Physiological Chemistry	1915	

TABLE 5.2   Loeb's nominators (*cont.*)

Number of nominations	Nominator	Discipline	first year	last year
1	Kaufmann, Jacob	Clinical Medicine	1920	
1	Laguesse, Edouard	Anatomy	1911	
1	Liebermann, Leo von	Hygiene	1912	
1	Long, John H	Chemistry	1912	
1	Lubarsch, Otto	Pathology	1919	
1	Maximow, Alexander A.	Histology	1914	
1	Meltzer, Samuel J.	Physiology	1913	
1	Meyer, Hans H.	Pharmacology	1912	
1	Michelson, Albert A.	Physics	1909	
1	Münsterberg, Hugo	Experimental Psychology	1901	
1	Osborne, Oliver T.	Therapeutics	1911	
1	Pavlov, Ivan P.	Physiology	1909	
1	Rauber, August	Anatomy	1909	
1	Richards, Alfred N.	Pharmacology	1913	
1	Sabin, Florence R.	Histology	1924	
1	Schamberg, Jay F.	Dermatology	1922	
1	Schultze, Bernhard	Gynecology	1912	
1	Senator, Hermann	Internal Medicine	1910	
1	Smith, Alexander	General Chemistry	1909	
1	Strahl, Hans	Anatomy	1911	
1	Swain, Henry L.	Laryngology	1911	
1	Weiss, Otto	Physiology	1919	
1	Winterstein, Hans	Physiology	1924	
1	Zuntz, Nathan	Zoophysiology	1919	
1	Zunz, Edgard	Pharmacology	1924	

a   Some data from Fangerau 2010 had to be corrected in view of the files instead of the database.

Ewald's nephew Wolfgang Felix – via his uncle – was able to become Loeb's assistant in 1912.[39] Ewald had been Friedrich Goltz's assistant and deputy when Loeb worked in Strassburg during the late 1880s with Goltz. Whereas the two

39   Loeb Papers, LC, Box Ewald.

had difficulties with each other during these years – at least from Loeb's side –[40] it seems that this did not affect Ewald's evaluation of Loeb negatively.

We do not know whether Loeb activated this network of colleagues in order to be nominated, however, in a contemporary comment, Jöns Johansson, who was asked to review Loeb's candidacy, noticed the relatively high number of nominations, some of which were received at the same time. Besides the attention for Loeb's work, Johansson attributed this phenomenon to 'advertisement' ('reklam') that had been made in favor of Loeb.[41] It remains unclear whether Johansson is alluding to the press reports on the artificial parthenogenesis experiment or to an advertisement for nominating Loeb within the scientific community. Simultaneously, Loeb also had colleagues to whom he had a close relationship who did not nominate him, although they had the chance of doing so. Wilhelm Roux, for example, who considered Loeb to be a close ally for his own research programme and who supported him on other occasions, never nominated him, although he had been invited to put forward a Nobel candidate.[42]

Evaluations by the Nobel Committee

The yearbooks in the Nobel Archive show that Loeb was considered a strong candidate. The Nobel committee completed four special investigations (1906, 1909, and two in 1917) by four different evaluators to determine his eligibility. The candidates on the shortlist were assessed, a process that was usually conducted by a member of the Nobel Committee and consisted of a description and evaluation of their research in question. Some reviewers also discussed the candidate's role in the scientific community by elucidating his or her competitors. Loeb's studies were analysed by a histologist in 1906 (Emil Holmgren) and a pharmacologist in 1909 (Karl Mörner). In 1917 two statements of a physiologist (Jöns Johansson) and an anatomist (Erik Müller) can be found in the files for the same year – a rare case.

1906 Evaluation by E. Holmgren

In 1906, Loeb received only one nomination together with Ernest Overton by Justus Gaule, for his work on artificial parthenogenesis and heterogeneous

---

40   Pauly 1987, 41.
41   Yearbook 1917 (Nobel Archive).
42   Halling, Hansson, Fangerau 2018.

hybridisation. Gaule also mentioned a previous nomination and stated that Loeb deserved the Prize now even more than four years before. In the same year, Loeb's German counterpart Max Verworn was also nominated by the pathologist Johannes Orth for his work on general physiology. Loeb and Verworn had at the beginning of their careers worked on similar topics, but later began to differ in research style and questions. Above all, Verworn disregarded Loeb's radical mechanistic standpoint while Loeb accused Verworn of an unsound holistic standpoint based on methods of comparative, descriptive morphology. Both were part of a larger scientific dispute among biologists who on the one hand considered themselves to represent a new kind of experimental biology (epitomised in characters like the founder of *developmental mechanics* Wilhelm Roux), as opposed to on the other hand traditional morphology.[43] Additionally, Loeb and Verworn saw themselves both as entrepreneurs of a new general physiology – Loeb concentrating on chemistry and mechanism, Verworn concentrating on the organic cell and conditionalism. They competed for influence in the same scientific arena, separated only by the Atlantic Ocean.

In that year Verworn did not make it to the shortlist.[44] Nevertheless, the 'morphologists' (as Loeb called them in his correspondence and books) represented by Verworn and Oscar and Richard Hertwig indirectly played a role against Loeb in the 1906 report. The first Nobel Committee report on Loeb was written in 1906 by the histologist Emil Holmgren, with a focus on artificial parthenogenesis.[45] According to Holmgren, Loeb's research on this matter was not really original, since other scholars before him had succeeded, through modifications of seawater, in affecting both fertilised and unfertilised eggs of the sea urchins and their further development. In the introduction of his 13-page report, Holmgren listed a few predecessors in this field, such as Oscar Hertwig, Éduard van Beneden, Eduard Strasburger, Theodor Boveri, Wilhelm Pfitzner, Friedrich Weismann, Samuel Steen Maxwell, as well as 'Richard Hertwig[,] [...] the first one to demonstrate unquestionable divisions of unfertilized eggs triggered by changes in the medium's chemical composition'. Holmgren appreciated that Loeb could drive unfertilised egg cells to division. However, the conclusions of this research were, in Holmgren's view, far-fetched and illusionary, only acknowledged by scientists far away from 'biological research branches':

---

43   Allen 1978.
44   On Loeb and Verworn as well as their animosity see Fangerau 2012; Pauly 1987, 84f.
45   Yearbook 1906 (Nobel Archive), Holmgren.

It is ridiculous to believe that an exclusively biological process like fertilization would only rely on physical-chemical processes. [...] How can Loeb argue, that fertilization only is a physical-chemical process?

Not surprisingly, Holmgren concluded that he could not recommend Loeb for the Nobel Prize. The debate he referred to had been triggered by Oscar Hertwig, when he in 1905 denied the importance of Loeb's work. For Hertwig the union of the egg's and the sperm's nuclear substances was the essential element in fertilisation. For Loeb this was a misunderstanding of the process itself which he attributed to the actions of ions.[46] For several years, the two of them fought a public dispute. A few years later, on 6 January 1911, Holmgren nominated Oscar Hertwig, who had rather strong scientific ties to Sweden for his work on fertilisation. Hertwig was elected fellow of the Royal Swedish Academy of Sciences in 1903 and he received an honorary doctorate at the University of Uppsala in 1907.[47] As an argument, Holmgren described Loeb as 'significantly inferior' to Hertwig. Loeb had clearly belonged to the wrong network in this case. From Loeb's perspective, Holmgren was – as a supporter of Hertwig – a very unfortunate reviewer.

1909 Evaluation by K. Mörner

The physiologist Mörner had a more positive tone in his 1909 report. That year, Loeb's nominations had reached a peak of ten. Loeb had just published a summarising book on his artificial parthenogenesis in German.[48] Furthermore, he had received a call to the university of Budapest – publicly discussed in various media:[49] Emile de Grosz (no motivation), Felix Mesnil (who nominated Loeb together with Émile Roux for work on tropism, artificial parthenogenesis and the antagonistic action of salts), Albert A. Michelson (artificial parthenogenesis, heterogeneous hybridization), Ivan Pavlov (artificial parthenogenesis, tropism, dynamics of living matter), August Rauber (together with Theodor Boveri and August Weismann for the chemistry of fertilization), Alexander Smith (physiology), Julius Stieglitz (artificial parthenogenesis, heterogeneous hybridization), Franz Tangl (artificial parthenogenesis), August von Wassermann

---

46   Cremer 1985, 105–109.
47   https://www.uu.se/en/about-uu/traditions/prizes/honorary-doctorates/medicine (accessed March 1, 2019).
48   Loeb 1909.
49   Pauly 1987, Fangerau 2010.

(artificial parthenogenesis, chemistry of fertilization) and – in group VII – Alexander Koranyi (artificial parthenogenesis).

According to reviewer Mörner, Loeb's research activities had, over decades, been original, including his theories on artificial parthenogenesis. As for the latter however, Mörner was unsure whether Loeb was the first one to relate haemolysis, parthenogenesis and cytolysis. Mörner raised a priority question referring to a speech held the very same year, in 1909, by Svante Arrhenius in the Royal Swedish Academy of Sciences. In that speech, Arrhenius supposedly had stated that he had written a letter to Loeb and informed him of the supposed relation. However, Loeb states that he got the idea in 1904 when he tried to figure out why membrane cultivation did not take place at his original method of 'artificial parthenogenesis'.[50]

As for the question of whether Loeb was prize-worthy, Mörner wrote that it had been correct not to consider him for the 1901 Prize, but, as Mörner put it: 'a very significant change has taken place since then… His investigations are of great interest for our understanding of the development of the egg and of the fertilization'. Although Mörner felt that Loeb's ideas were 'tempting and spiritual', he did not give Loeb a full recommendation for two reasons. First, he thought that Loeb's theories needed to stand on a more solid ground. Second, he wrote that one should await the development of the 'individuals', who had been created by artificial parthenogenesis and that it would be of great importance to find out if his findings on sea-urchins also may apply to mammals.

At that time, Loeb's work on egg development was still controversial. And again, the Hertwig brothers stood in the way: 'Without any doubt, he has many admirers, and some of them are men with scientific authority'.[51] But, he also had, according to Mörner, opponents mostly among the morphologists. Mörner also reported the most recent critics against Loeb formulated by Oscar Hertwig in his study *Der Kampf um Kernfragen der Entwicklung und Vererbungslehre*.[52] Nevertheless, Mörner was not convinced that there really existed a substantial difference between Loeb's experimental approach, which he shared with developmental mechanics like Wilhelm Roux,[53] and methods fostered by, for example, the Hertwigs. In Mörner's opinion, the controversies could be explained by the fact that researchers tend to view their own methods as the most meaningful ones. Thus, both sides in that quarrel were 'somewhat

50   Yearbook 1909 (Nobel Archive), Mörner.
51   Yearbook 1909 (Nobel Archive), Mörner.
52   Hertwig 1909. See in particular the pages 109–113 about Loeb.
53   Halling, Fangerau, Hansson 2018.

one-sided'. Due to these quarrels, however, Mörner concluded not to propose Loeb for a Nobel Prize: 'Although I do not agree with Hertwig on this matter, I find it not yet reasonable to recommend Loeb for the Nobel Prize'.[54]

1917 Evaluation 1 by J. Johansson and Evaluation 2 by E. Müller

In 1917, the last time Loeb was considered for a report, he had been proposed by two colleagues from the RIMR. One short nomination was brought forward by the institute's director Simon Flexner, who stressed Loeb's work in the broad field of experimental biology. The other was from the biochemist Phoebus Levene, who singled out artificial parthenogenesis. A little bit too late (on the 3rd of February) a third nomination by the German serologist August von Wassermann reached the committee, in which he (referring to previous nominations) briefly nominated Loeb without further explanation. The reports were written by the physiologist Jöns Johansson and the anatomist Erik Müller, both from the Karolinska Institute.

As stated above, in 1917 Johansson found it remarkable that Loeb by then had been nominated quite often for the Nobel Prize. Loeb's greatest virtue, however, was the tenacity with which he pursued his ideas. Although Johansson admitted that Loeb's overviews of issues in the general physiology were as original as the contributions made by previous award-winning scientists, he raised objections against the conclusions and generalisations that Loeb had drawn from his findings. Although he expected that Loeb ultimately would succeed in completing his theory of the egg division process, it seemed to him that possibly other physiologists were more deserving, even if they were not among that year's candidates. Müller also confronted Loeb's discoveries and theoretical hypotheses, which he found hard to distinguish, with contradicting theories and rejections by other scientists like the French zoologist Yves Delage or the American embryologist Ralph S. Lillie. 'One must distinguish between Loeb's actual discoveries and his theoretical hypothesis', he wrote:

Even if we acknowledge Loeb's premise to understand development processes through chemistry, and if we admire his deductions, which strive to realize the alchemists dreamed objective: the synthesis of living matter, we must conclude, that his lysin-theory is not a clear-cut physical-chemical explanation of fertilization and parthenogenesis. [...] The

54   Yearbook 1909 (Nobel Archive), Mörner, 11.

French zoologist Yves Delage rejects Loeb's theory, as well as the American embryologist R.S. Lillie, who has seen Loeb's work at Woods Hole. Hence, it is easy to find opponents. Moreover, it is hard to combine Loeb's chemical theory with the findings of Albert P. Matthews on the one hand [to stir eggs of sea-urchins to start a parthenogenetic development], and with Bataillon's on the other.[55]

Eugène Bataillon (who in 1919 also nominated Loeb for the Nobel Prize) had in 1910 introduced a different method of producing artificial parthenogenesis which conformed to earlier observations on marine invertebrates. Loeb had changed the electrolyte environment of sea urchin eggs, Bataillon, by puncturing frogs' eggs with extremely fine needles, was able to bring about a division of the egg. Loeb subsequently took up the same method and at times was able to make the eggs develop into sexually mature frogs which closely resembled those raised in the normal manner. Nevertheless, Müller acknowledged Loeb's priority and his skills at transgressing disciplinary borders. He stated:

> It probably is universally recognized, that Loeb's demonstration of artificial parthenogenesis is a scientific discovery of premier rank. Loeb's priority is undeniable, even if we consider R. Hertwig's experiments on sea-urchins in 1895, or Morgan's in hypertonic seawater in 1896. Loeb has opened an entirely new research field, which has become one of the most important fields within physiological morphology. It is a great achievement that Loeb has been able to synthesize morphology and chemistry to one subject. He must be evaluated by experts in morphology and chemistry (in this evaluation, his work is viewed from a morphological standpoint, thus it is not complete). Having said that, to me personally it is of no doubt that Loeb deserves the Nobel Prize, even though I can understand if some would question this decision because of the discussion about the theoretical evidence of artificial parthenogenesis.[56]

In the closing remarks, however, Müller struck a deadly blow as he candidly wrote: 'If I compare Harrison with Loeb, I would vote in favour of Harrison because of the fact that his ground-breaking investigations were immediately recognized.' It seems as if there has been simply too much debate about Loeb's

---

55   Yearbook 1917 (Nobel Archive), Müller.
56   Yearbook 1917 (Nobel Archive), Müller.

controversial findings. The reviewers could not get themselves to award a prize against all the opposition.

Prize Discussions in the Nobel Committee 1917

Müller's reference to Harrison was due to the fact that Harrison was also shortlisted that very year. Harrison, who, by the way, had a friendly personal correspondence with Loeb (Fangerau 2010, 148f), had worked successfully on the culture of nerve fibre in vitro (Maienschein 1983). The following candidates made it – apart from Loeb – to the shortlist in 1906, 1909 and 1917. 1906: C. Golgi, R. Cajal, E. Overton, A. Bier, Ch. J. Finlay, H. Carter, A. Laveran, P. Ehrlich; 1909: E. Fischer, A. Bier, H. Quincke, V. Horsley, Th. Kocher, J. Bordet, R. Pfeiffer, Th. Smith; 1917: H. Gutzmann, B. Krönig, C. Eijkman, J. Bordet, W. Einthoven, R.G. Harrison.

Only on rare occasions were prize discussions brought to protocol. One of these exceptions is found is the yearbook of 1917, where single Nobel Committee members announced their opinion on the researchers on the short list. The physiologist Jöns Johansson did not see the shortlisted Willem Einthoven as a strong candidate, since he 'merely has developed an instrument'. As for Loeb, his work was interpreted to be of particularly large value, but the physical-chemical part was held not to be sufficiently investigated – he called for a further investigation: 'Thus, he shall not be proposed by the Committee this year either'.

As shown above, the Committee member Erik Müller was enthusiastic of Ross G. Harrison. In the nominations of Harrison, it was stated that he had placed fragments from frog embryos in a drop of clotted frog's lymph. Müller gave him a full recommendation and meant that his research was 'of great importance' and 'performed recently'. Although Müller's arguments mirrored the stipulations in Alfred Nobel's will, again, Jöns Johansson was cautious: 'I am not convinced that Harrison is the best candidate and therefore suggest, that no Prize shall be awarded this year.'[57] Johansson's proposal lost by one vote (Müller, Lennmalm, Sundberg for R. Harrison, Johansson and Westermark for no Prize). Thus, the Committee nominated Harrison with the motivation: 'for his discovery of the development of the nerve fibres by independent growth from cells outside the organism.'[58]

---

57   Yearbook 1917 (Nobel Archive).
58   Yearbook 1917 (Nobel Archive).

However, the Nobel Assembly did not agree and chose not to award the Prize in 1917. That was not the only occasion on which the Nobel Assembly did not follow the recommendation of the Nobel Committee. As Ragnar Björk has shown, the Committee even twice proposed Carl Neuberg, but could not get support from the Assembly.[59]

Conclusion

Loeb died in 1924 without a Nobel Prize after having received almost 100 nominations. Had Loeb been a wrong candidate? Some features in his research, his publication style and his self-promotion seem to have made him appear 'second best'. Taking the reports of the referees into account, his combination of methods seems to have been an asset and an obstacle. Yet, he did not fit into the right shelf. Although he was nominated for many of his fields of work, he was considered in the evaluations only for his controversially discussed 'artificial parthenogenesis'. His synthetic approach linking morphology and chemistry was appreciated as innovative but considered as far-fetched. All four evaluations lamented the lack of a proof of concept. Additionally, his priority was doubted. Although his concepts seemed to be too visionary on the one hand, his research itself was on the other hand presented as mainstream research in line with many other colleagues who in the end contradicted his conclusions. Here, a personal feature of Loeb might have played a role: he presented himself as an archetypical mechanist and fought against any other stance. He also was an ardent reductionist, confronting with pleasure his position with any grand theory like Darwinism or vitalism which, according to his view, did not take the physio-chemical basis of life adequately into account.[60] This uncompromising, rigid and sometimes personally intransigent stance was indirectly remarked when his works were contrasted to those of Hertwig. Therefore, it seems as if Loeb had made too many enemies in the end to be awarded the Prize.

Taking the high number of nominations for Loeb into account our study reveals that numbers did not count for the Nobel committee. On the contrary, as Johansson's remark on the advertisement can be understood, the committee was not impressed by the nomination politics obviously put forward by some scientific circles. The sheer number of nominations and the frequent nominations of Loeb by RIMR fellows, together with the fact that some of

---

59   Björk 2001.
60   Pauly 1987, Fangerau 2010.

the nominations were extremely short, call to mind a general observation Liljestrand expressed in his book from 1963. 'Frequently', he wrote,

> several members of the same faculty propose a common candidate – in most cases a fellow-countryman, who is sometimes, moreover, one of their own faculty colleagues – and they usually do it, either in a joint statement, or in personal letters which in content vary very little from each other. This procedure is probably due to the erroneous assumption that the prize-distributing bodies will be impressed and influenced in proportion to the number of supporters a candidate has among those officially invited to submit nominations. This idea has become so common that it has often been possible to predict with a fair degree of accuracy, even before opening a letter to the Committee, the name of the candidate it has supported.[61]

After the First World War, the pattern of Loeb's nominations slightly changed and inclined even more in the direction observed by Liljestrand. The disintegration of Loeb's European roots resulted in more than 50% of his post-war nominations stemming from Americans. Whereas his German nominators held their pre-war share, the Hungarian nominations from Budapest for example, which had contributed much to his nomination statistics before the war, declined substantially. Loeb now had become an American candidate.[62]

This external image was also reflected in his self-image. During the war, Loeb's critical standpoint towards European (science) politics in general and German (science) politics in particular intensified. He was shocked by the War and the disintegration of international science. In his public writings and in his correspondence – for example with Svante Arrhenius – he strongly expressed his disapproval of scientists engaging in the war. He could not understand why his former friends like Wilhelm Ostwald or Charles Richet (one of his nominators) participated in the propaganda for their respective countries.[63] During the War, he became an ardent antagonist of German imperialism which he also partly attributed in his writings to the morphological school of biology. His argument was that the German idea of racial superiority, which nurtured

---

61 Liljestrand 1962, 149f.
62 Nevertheless, he also suffered from anti-German, anti-Semitic tendencies in the USA. In 1922 he wrote to Flexner: 'Since I was born in Germany my participation in the meeting [a meeting by the Bunsen-Gesellschaft in Germany] might be utilized by the jingoes and the antisemitic crowd in the American Universities to make trouble for me.' (Loeb to Flexner 02.06.1922, American Philosophical Society Archives, Flexner Papers).
63 Reingold and Reingold 1981, 224f.

the war, was fostered by morphologically oriented biologists and that a mechanistic standpoint would have at least not contributed to this idea.[64] Loeb was
puzzled by the fact that his former friends favoured the German case. Even his
first nominator, Hugo Münsterberg, a German patriot himself suffering from
the deterioration of the German-American relationship, was accused by him
of 'irresponsibly' preaching the 'spirit of brutal egotism'[65] nurturing the war.

In his fight for politics through science Loeb himself in the end intended
to include the Nobel Prize. He supported colleagues in receiving it, but at the
same time he – disappointed by the First World War – suggested to use Nobel's money rather for the internationalization and democratization of science
than for further Prizes. Without knowing of Münsterberg's earlier nomination,
which seems to contradict his own feelings towards Münsterberg 15 years later,
he expressed similar ideas towards the danger of German scientific organization when he wrote to Svante Arrhenius in March 1918:

> I feel very strongly the necessity of saving the world from the subtle influ-
> ence of German scientific teaching and scientific literary organization.
> [...] It seems to me that you in Sweden should take the first step by utilis-
> ing the money for the Nobel Prizes for the equipment of your research
> institutions. [...] with the impoverishment following the war, with the
> necessity of providing research institutions outside of Germany to save
> the world from their philosophy of organization, brutality, anti-Semitism,
> and the Lord knows what else, it becomes imperative that we do every-
> thing to prevent the victory of the Germans over the minds of the coming
> generations. It seems to me that it becomes a duty of the friends of liberty
> to insist that the money for the Nobel prizes for one thing should at least
> for the next twenty-five or fifty years be utilized in building up research
> in Sweden [...].[66]

Definitely, Loeb's candidacy was a near miss, but finally he indirectly stayed
involved in the Prize circus after the war and even after his death in 1924. He
succeeded on other levels. It is as if Julius Richard Ewald's prognosis given in
one nomination had become true. Ewald wrote: '... Loeb's works are ... like a

---

64   Fangerau 2009; Fangerau 2007.
65   Loeb to Sarton 16.12.1916, Houghton Library, Harvard Sarton bMS Am 1803 (950), see
      (Fangerau 2010, 108).
66   Loeb to Arrhenius 11.03.1918, Loeb papers, LC, see (Fangerau 2010, 116f). See similar letters
      Loeb to Arrhenius printed in Reingold and Reingold 1981.

cheque, which is paid in the future, compared to the safe value of cash'.[67] Some of the colleagues he actively supported received the Prize in the years to come (for example Otto Meyerhof in 1922, Charles Sherrington in 1932, his former assistant John Howard Northrop in 1946 (for chemistry)). His reductionist research approach (although in a mechanistic shape already contested by his contemporaries) was to have a lasting influence on the life sciences in the United States.[68]

Acknowledgment

Files on Loeb in the Nobel Prize archive were kindly provided by the Nobel Committee for Physiology or Medicine. All translations from Swedish and German to English were done by the authors.

Bibliography

Allen, G. 1978. *Life Science in the Twentieth Century*. Cambridge, MA: Cambridge University Press

Allen, G. 1978. *Thomas Hunt Morgan: The Man and His Science*. Princeton: Princeton University Press.

Anon. 1903. "The Nobel Prizes". *Boston Medical and Surgical Journal* 149 (20): 554–555.

Anon. 1904. "Credit Due American Investigators". *JAMA* 42 (1): 39.

Anon. 1905. "Our Attitude Toward The Nobel Prizes". *JAMA* 44 (15): 1201.

Björk, R. 2001. "Inside the Nobel Committee on Medicine: Prize Competition Procedures 1901–1950 and the Fate of Carl Neuberg". *Minerva* 39(4): 393–408.

Bucchi, M. 2015. "Norms, Competition and Visibility in Contemporary Science: The Legacy of Robert K. Merton". *Journal of Classic Sociology* 15: 233–252.

Cremer, T. 1985. Von der Zellenlehre zur Chromosomentheorie. Naturwissenschaftliche Erkenntnis und Theorienwechsel in der frühen Zell- und Vererbungsforschung. Berlin, Heidelberg: Springer.

Enke, U. 2018. "'Der erste zu sein.' – Über den ersten Medizinnobelpreis für Emil von Behring im Jahr 1901". In *Der Nobelpreis. Konstruktion von Exzellenz zu Beginn des 20. Jahrhunderts (Berichte zur Wissenschaftsgeschichte* 41 (1)), edited by T. Halling; H. Fangerau; N. Hansson, 19–46. Weinheim: Wiley-VCH.

---

67   Yearbook 1909 (Nobel Archive).
68   Pauly 1987.

Fangerau, H. 2007. "Biology and War". *History and Philosophy of the Life Sciences* 29 (4): 395–427.

Fangerau, H. 2009. "From Mephistopheles to Iesajah: Jacques Loeb, Science and Modernism". *Social Studies of Science* 39: 229–256.

Fangerau, H. 2010. *Spinning the Scientific Web: Jacques Loeb (1859–1924) und sein Programm einer internationalen biomedizinischen Grundlagenforschung*. Berlin: Akademie Verlag.

Fangerau, H. 2012. "Monism, Racial Hygiene, and National Socialism". In *Monism. Science, Philosophy, Religion, and the History of a Worldview*, edited by T. Weir, 223–247. New York: Palgrave.

Fangerau, H. and Müller, I. 2005. "Loeb, Jacques". In *Germany and the Americas. Culture, Politics, and History (Transatlantic Relations Series)*, edited by T. Adam, 691–692. Santa Barbara (CA): ABC-CLIO.

Halling, T.; Fangerau, H.; Hansson, N. (eds.). 2018. *Der Nobelpreis. Konstruktion von Exzellenz zu Beginn des 20. Jahrhunderts (Berichte zur Wissenschaftsgeschichte 41 (1))*. Weinheim: Wiley-VCH.

Halling, T.; Hansson, N.; Fangerau H. 2018. "'Prisvärdig' Forschung? Wilhelm Roux und sein Programm der Entwicklungsmechanik". In *Der Nobelpreis. Konstruktion von Exzellenz zu Beginn des 20. Jahrhunderts (Berichte zur Wissenschaftsgeschichte 41 (1))*, edited by T. Halling; H. Fangerau; N. Hansson, 73–97. Weinheim: Wiley-VCH.

Hansson, N. and Schlich, T. 2014. "'A Life Dedicated to True Science': Eduard Pflüger and the Nobel Prize for Physiology or Medicine". *Pflügers Archiv – European Journal of Physiology* 466 (11): 2021–2024.

Hollingsworth, J.R. 2004. "Institutionalizing Excellence in Biomedical Research: The Case of The Rockefeller University". In *Creating a Tradition of Biomedical Research. Contributions to the History of the Rockefeller University*, edited by D.H. Stapleton, 17–63. New York: Rockefeller University Press.

Liljestrand, G. 1962. "The Prize in Physiology or Medicine". In *Nobel: The Man and His Prizes*, edited by H. Schück et al., 135–316. Amsterdam: Elsevier.

Loeb, J. 1899. "On the Nature of the Process of Fertilization and the Artificial Production of Normal Larvae (Plutei) from the Unfertilized Eggs of Sea Urchins". *American Journal of Physiology* 3: 135–138.

Loeb, J. 1909. "Die chemische Entwicklungserregung des tierischen Eies: Künstliche Parthenogenese". Berlin: Springer

Luttenberger, F. 1996. "Excellence and Chance: The Nobel Prize Case of E. von Behring and E. Roux". *History of Philosophy of the Life Sciences* 18: 225–239.

Maienschein, J. 1983. "Experimental Biology in Transition: Harrison's Embryology, 1895–1910." *Studies in History of Biology* 6: 107–127.

Merton, R.K. 1968. "The Matthew Effect in Science". *Science* 159 (3810): 56–63.

Naylor, C.D. and Bell, J.I. 2015. "On the Recognition of Global Excellence in Medical Research". *JAMA*. 314 (11): 1125–1126.

Pauly, P.J. 1987. *Controlling Life: Jacques Loeb and the Engineering Ideal in Biology*. New York: Oxford University Press.

Rasmussen, C.T. and Tilman, R. 1998. *Jacques Loeb: His Science and Social Activism and Their Philosophical Foundations* (Memoirs of the American Philosophical Society 229). Philadelphia: American Philosophical Society.

Reingold, N. and Reingold, I. (eds.). 1981. *A Documentary History, 1900–1939* (Chicago History of Science and Medicine). Chicago: University of Chicago Press.

Turney, J. 1995. "Life in the Laboratory: Public Responses to Experimental Biology." *Public understanding of science* 4 (2): 153–176.

Whitley, R. 2000. *The intellectual and Social Organization of the Sciences*. Oxford: Oxford University Press.

CHAPTER 6

Defining 'Cutting-edge' Excellence: Awarding Nobel Prizes (or not) to Surgeons

Nils Hansson, David S. Jones and Thomas Schlich

[T]he Nobel award casts a glow of pride over all those associated with the recipient, through their field of science, their professions, or their institutions.[1]

As I walked across the stage to meet King Gustav IV as he approached me from the opposite side, the whole experience seemed like a fairy tale. Here I was – a clinical doctor, a surgeon whose professional life was devoted primarily to taking care of patients – receiving the world's most prestigious scientific prize.[2]

These two quotes by surgeons, the first by Francis D. Moore and the second by Joseph Murray (Nobel laureate in physiology or medicine in 1990), show the extent to which surgeons consider the Nobel Prize to be the strongest symbol of scientific excellence in our time – this despite the fact that it has rarely been awarded to surgeons. Given the significance of the award, it is not surprising that its effects on the scientific community have inspired burgeoning scholarship by historians of medicine and science.[3] The Nobel Prize archives in Sweden, made accessible for each year after a fifty-year delay (e.g., the records for 1969 will become available in 2019) offer scholars the opportunity to peer behind the curtain and study the selection process for Nobel laureates. Historians have payed particular attention to the Nobel committee's special investigations to reconstruct how the nominees were evaluated and a few were chosen to become laureates. In this chapter, we will focus not on the evaluation process but on the Nobel Prize nominations themselves in order to examine the standards of excellence, originality and credit used in and for surgery. What accomplishments were emphasized when a surgeon was nominated? When possible we also examine the jury investigations to study the mechanics of the

---

1   Moore 1995, 321–322.
2   Murray 2001, 221.
3   Zuckerman 1977; Friedman 2001; Crawford 2002.

decision-making process and ascertain the arguments for or against recognition of particular surgical achievements.

Nobel Prizes for the development of surgical procedures as such are relatively rare. To date, only four laureates are obvious: Theodor Kocher in 1909 'for his work on the physiology, pathology and surgery of the thyroid gland', Alexis Carrel in 1912 'in recognition of his work on vascular suture and the transplantation of blood vessels and organs', António Egas Moniz in 1949 'for his discovery of the therapeutic value of leucotomy in certain psychoses', and Joseph Murray in 1990 'for discoveries concerning organ and cell transplantation in the treatment of human disease' (official motivations by the Nobel Committee).[4]

However, the actual laureates represent only the tip of the iceberg. The nominations for the award are much more numerous. The first Nobel Prize was awarded in 1901. Nominations for surgeons soon followed. William Mayo, for instance, one of the founders of the acclaimed Mayo Clinic, was nominated by surgeon Albert John Ochsner in 1909:

> The motive for this proposal lies in the fact that through his incessant scientific work, Dr. Mayo has increased the usefulness of surgical methods to so great an extent during the past ten years that the surgical profession from all parts of the World has followed his teaching both by visiting his clinics and by studying the great number of scientific monographs which he has produced to such an extent that virtually the entire surgical world has been able to increase its efficiency in the treatment of the sick.[5]

Lord Joseph Lister received a nomination the following year, having 'done more for the good of humanity than any other member of the medical profession of all countries at present living'.[6]

The rhetoric in these two examples is typical of Nobel nominations in their characterization of surgical candidates as scientific heroes, geniuses, world-leaders, and influential men of action.[7] Following the lead of recent

---

4 Schlich 2007; However, there have been several Nobel laureates, who were trained as surgeons who did not receive the Prize for the development of a surgical procedure, but for something else: Allvar Gullstrand 1911, Robert Bárány 1914, Frederick Banting 1929, Alexander Fleming 1945, Walter Rudolf Hess 1949, Werner Forssmann 1956 and Charles Huggins 1966.
5 Yearbook 1909 (Nobel Archive).
6 Yearbook 1910 (Nobel Archive).
7 Lawrence 1992.

historiography on scientific merit,[8] we look at excellence not as an inherent quality of an achievement or of a person, but as the result of a process of attribution. Nobel nominations constitute ideal source material to shed light on such processes. They provide us with information on the reputation of some of the best-known surgeons in the United States and Europe – arguably the main centers of surgical research during the 20th century[9] – including William Halsted, Ferdinand Sauerbruch, August Bier, Jacques Louis Reverdin, Erwin Payr, John B Murphy, Victor Horsley, René Leriche, and Harvey Cushing, to mention just a few. As these examples indicate, the lion's share of all nominees within this category were men. Only a small fraction of the candidates with links to surgery were female, such as Alice Bernheim for her work on the function of the parathyroid glands and Helen B. Taussig (a cardiologist) for the Blalock-Taussig shunt (see below). Our account does not aim at revealing bias and partiality in the selection process, criticizing the decisions of the Nobel committee, or giving instructions on how to play the system. Instead, we use the nominations and evaluations as a window to look into the mechanisms of recognition in medicine and science. With this, we hope to obtain insight into how excellence is attributed and how surgery, in particular, has been discussed in the context of scientific excellence in the twentieth century.

Surgery is a particularly interesting field to study for this purpose because, as Jacalyn Duffin points out, '[no] medical heroes have enjoyed greater prestige than the surgeons of the late nineteenth and early twentieth centuries, surgeons who devised daring and previously inconceivable responses to internal pathology'.[10] However, the lines of separation between surgery and internal medicine were often indistinct in the twentieth century, with both collaborations and overlap with other specialties. This makes it sometimes difficult to determine if a Nobel Prize candidate should be categorized as a surgeon. Topics such as hyperthyroidism, or certain neurological and psychiatric diagnoses, moved between the fields of surgery and medicine. The 1909 Nobel Prize for the surgeon Theodor Kocher, for instance, underlined his achievement in the physiology, pathology and surgery of the thyroid gland. For the purposes of this study, we have decided to view all candidates as surgeons if they were at least listed once as surgeons under the headline 'therapy/surgery' in the yearbooks of the Nobel Prize committee. The yearbooks were divided into sections for different thematic and disciplinary areas. Many specialists appeared under

---

8   Jordanova 1995; Woolgar 1976; Reverby and Rosner 2004; More specifically on surgery, see
       Frampton 2016.
9   Schlich 2016.
10   Duffin 2010, 266.

'therapy/surgery' headline during the first half of the 20th century, not only general surgeons but also gynecologists, orthopedists, otolaryngologists, anesthesiologists, and urologists.[11] In some instance, a specific individual was categorized as a surgeon in one yearbook and as a physiologist, neurologist, or pharmacologist in another. Harvey Cushing, for example, was evaluated by the Nobel Committee in different years by a physiologist, a surgeon, a neurosurgeon, a pharmacologist, a pathologist, and a neurologist. This disciplinary ambiguity was also mirrored in Nobel nominations. William Cone, for instance, wrote in his nomination letter that his Montreal colleague Walter Penfield 'is internationally recognized by neurosurgeons as a leader in clinical neurology and in the surgery of the nervous system'.[12] In such cases, we have 'followed' the candidate in the different groups 'physiology' and 'therapy/surgery', once they had been grouped under 'surgery/therapy' even if they were switched into a different category later on.

Considering the rareness of Nobel Prizes in surgery, one might wonder if there was something about surgery as a field that made it less suitable for a prize. Alfred Nobel's will of 1895 provides little specific guidance. It stipulated merely that the prizes should be given to 'those who, during the preceding year, shall have conferred the greatest benefit to mankind'. Surgeons have certainly made innovations. They have opened up new domains of therapeutic action. Many patients have benefited. So what is the problem? Is it that surgeons develop techniques or devices instead of discovering new facts about nature? Is it that it is rarely possible to identify the one, two, or three people who deserve the prize for a particular innovation in surgery? In the following, we will discuss some possible reasons. Our main focus lies on transplant surgeons, cardiac surgeons, and brain surgeons. They represent three fields of surgery that received much attention from nominators and the Nobel Prize committee over certain periods of time.

Transplant Surgery

In the late nineteenth century, the idea that complex internal diseases could be successfully treated by replacing a failing organ was still met with skepticism. Thus the Amsterdam surgeon Otto Lanz wrote in 1897 that one should not make light of the idea of organ transplants even though the method looks like

---

11   Hansson 2018; Hansson, Fangerau, Tuffs et al. 2017; Hansson, Halling, Moll et al. 2017; Hansson, Halling, Fangerau 2016; Hansson 2015.
12   Yearbook 1958 (Nobel Archive).

it comes straight from 'a quack's handbook'.[13] This was a point in time when transplant surgery was just starting to be seen as a promising strategy for the rational, science-based treatment of disease. In its connection to experimental science and its almost utopian vision of replaceability, it quickly became the epitome of the promises held by modern medicine.

The Nobel laureate Theodor Kocher was crucially involved in discovering the concept of organ replacement. In 1882, he performed the first organ transplant in the modern sense of replacing an organ to treat a complex internal disease when he implanted thyroid tissue into one of his patients to alleviate the symptoms occurring after a total thyroidectomy. This first transplant became the model for numerous experiments and therapeutic operations in organ transplantation and eventually led to the acceptance of the concept.[14] As Ulrich Tröhler has shown, Kocher was nominated at least six times for the Prize starting in 1907, before he became the first surgeon to receive it. In his Nobel speech, Kocher mentioned the potential implications of his discovery of the function of the thyroid gland for transplantation as a new revolutionary mode of surgical therapy of internal diseases.[15]

The Nobel Prize for Alexis Carrel in 1912 was officially awarded to him in recognition of his suture technique that resulted in reliable vascular anastomoses without the formation of blood clots. The method allowed repairing injuries of the larger blood vessels, but, from the start, Carrel also aimed at using it to facilitate organ transplantation, as vascular reattachment was essential for the success of most transplanted organs. Among surgeons at the time, Carrel's techniques were widely perceived as a breakthrough that would make organ transplants clinically viable.

Interestingly enough, Carrel was only nominated a few times, the first time in 1910 by Carl Beck with a short motivation: 'Thanking you for the honor conferred upon me I beg to submit the name of Alexis Carrel of the Rockefeller Institute of New York for his work on Surgery of the blood vessels'.[16] Other nominations also mentioned his experimental work on new ways of transplanting animal tissue, and on its survival outside the body and its behavior after transplantation into a different animal, including Carrel's attempts at growing adult animal and human tissue on artificial culture media in the context of cancer research.

In the first and last special investigation on behalf of the Nobel committee in 1912, the reviewer, surgeon Jules Åkerman, envisioned a huge potential for

---

13   Schlich 2010.
14   Schlich 2010.
15   Tröhler 2013; Tröhler 1984.
16   Yearbook 1910 (Nobel Archive).

organ transplants using the vascular suture. He thought that allotransplants and autotransplants were especially promising. However, Carrel's numerous experiments on transplantation of the kidney had revealed that the interactions of the organ and of its host needed more intensive research. At this point, scientists had not identified the phenomenon of transplant rejection. Instead they thought that transplant failure was due to technical problems, which could be fixed by further improvement of the surgical procedure. Organ transplantation seemed to be within immediate grasp of contemporary surgeons. The Nobel committee settled on the surgeon Alexis Carrel with the following justification: 'For his works on vascular suture, the transplantation of blood vessels and organs as well as the culture and growth of tissues in vitro'.[17] Before the award ceremony the last passage on tissue culture was dropped to avoid a scientific priority dispute with other researchers, so that the final motivation ran as follows: 'in recognition of his work on vascular suture and the transplantation of blood vessels and organs'.[18]

Carrel received a diploma, a medal, and $39,000 (corresponds today to a value of $950,000), but the international renown was probably more important, as one commentator has suggested: 'If ever Carrel had been an ugly duckling, he was certainly now a swan. His laboratories on York Avenue became increasingly a place of pilgrimage'.[19] Carrel's award was considered the first American Nobel Prize in physiology or medicine, although Carrel was a French citizen. In reaction, leading journals underlined the outstanding reputation of the award and at the same appreciated the choice made by the Nobel Committee. Soon after the prize had been announced, the Lancet emphasized Carrel's 'wonderful manipulative dexterity, his extraordinary originality', and that the honour 'does not come as a surprise'.[20] Similarly, the *Boston Medical and Surgical Journal* (in 1928 renamed *New England Journal of Medicine*) stated that Carrel now 'takes his place formally and officially among the great ones of the earth by the award of the Nobel Prize'.[21] The *New York Times* presented Carrel's work as a 'miracle in surgery'.[22]

Our examination of the discussions about the Nobel Prize for Alexis Carrel in 1912 suggests that the Prize was meant to be a reward for a visionary new treatment strategy. Transplantation was seen as a promising technological fix for various complex internal diseases. Excellence in medicine was in this case

---

17   Yearbook 1912 (Nobel Archive).
18   Yearbook 1912 (Nobel Archive).
19   Le Vay 1996, 93.
20   Lancet 1912.
21   Anon. NEJM 1912.
22   Anon. NYT 1912.

not a matter of being a first-class researcher or surgeon, but rather measured by the potential impact of the innovation at hand. This was above all what made a new technique or new knowledge attractive for the Nobel Prize committee. Transplantation was clearly seen as a promising route towards the medicine of the future, embodying the potential of a straightforward surgical solution to complex medical problems.[23] It was the vision of a revolutionary and at the same time plausible breakthrough in medicine that motivated the jury.

Cardiac Surgery

If one asked surgeons about the most dramatic developments in medicine in the twentieth century, cardiac surgery would certainly be on their list. Historians of medicine would probably agree. Surgeons had long been frightened of operating on the heart, as seen with the famous – and possibly apocryphal – warning of Theodor Billroth in 1882 ('Any surgeon who wishes to preserve the respect of his colleagues would never attempt to operate on the heart').[24] The high caution towards this organ lasted until the 1940s, when it gave way to extraordinary surgical bravado and progress through the 1960s, embodied in first attempts to repair congenital heart disease through the drama of open heart surgery, heart transplantation, and artificial hearts.

Many of the key figures of this era were nominated for the Nobel Prize, including Evarts Graham for his work on thoracic surgery; Robert Gross, Clarence Crafoord, and Russel Brock for their work on vascular malformations; Alfred Blalock and Helen Taussig, for the famous 'blue baby' operation; and John Gibbon and Walt Lillehei for the heart-lung machines that made open heart surgery possible. Non-invasive procedures on the heart by thoracic surgeons also received some attention. In 1963, U.S. cardiac surgeon Claude S. Beck nominated William B Kouwenhoven, James R Jude, and Guy Knickerbocker for their work on closed chest massage for patients who suffered cardiac arrest. Beck used the opportunity to criticize the exaggerated attention paid to open heart surgery:

> This contribution makes it possible to reverse the fatal heart attack outside the hospital, without opening the chest, without getting dirty and it

---

23   To date no fewer than eight Nobel Prizes were awarded to scientists and doctors who worked on some aspect of transplant medicine.

24   Billroth, quoted in: Monagan and Williams 2007, 13; some authors doubt the authenticity of this quotation. See Blatchford and Rehn 1985.

can be done by laymen [...]Society is heart-conscious – receptive to high recognition. Surgical operations on the heart are dramatic. They are technical, involve the use of the hands and to a lesser extent medical science. Surgical developments are important but they are primarily technical and their import is limited to the individual patient.[25]

The Nobel Prize nominations indicate the diversity of innovation that nominators valued. Sometimes they praised originality. Sometimes they highlighted fundamental contributions to surgery and to medical science. In other cases, they credited surgeons with opening up whole new areas of surgical therapeutics. For instance, when LM Freeman nominated Gibbon in 1959, he argued that

the tremendous strides made in the field of cardiovascular surgery overwhelm all other developments. In attempting to determine the reason for the remarkable achievement, many contributions come to one's mind. However, there appears to be a common denominator from which all of the advances stem. This is the pump oxygenator apparatus and to its first useful adaptation in both animals and man credit goes to John Gibbon.[26]

The heart was obviously an organ that elicited respect and fascination. The new ability to operate on it successfully was widely described as a revolution worthy of particular appreciation. This shows up clearly in the wording of the more than forty nominations for Alfred Blalock and Helen Taussig for their development of surgical repairs of congenital heart disease. A 1955 nomination, for example, argued that Blalock has had 'a profound influence throughout the world of investigators, clinicians and surgeons to attack these problems from different angles for the improvement of mankind'.[27] Despite this enthusiasm, the Nobel committee never awarded the pair a prize. It requested confidential expert opinions on Blalock and Taussig, a brief examination of their case in 1947, and thorough special investigations in 1949, 1954, and 1956. The committee had different concerns in different years. In 1954 the two heart specialists were critiqued for having provided only palliation with their new techniques, and not a cure of the underlying disease. Timing proved to be important in this

---

25 Yearbook 1963 (Nobel Archive); Nomination for W.B. Kouwenhoven, James R Jude, Guy Knickerbocker by Claude S. Beck, Cleveland/Ohio (1963). Clarence Crafoord evaluated them on behalf of the Nobel committee in 1963. He did not view them as prize-worthy.

26 Yearbook 1959 (Nobel Archive).

27 Hansson and Schlich 2015a.

case as well. In 1956 the reviewer's concern was that their technique was no longer in use, having been superseded by a series of refinements. It now looked like a pioneer method of historical importance only.

As the Nobel archives become available for the late 1960s and 1970s, it will become possible to see how the committee responded to two other crucial innovations in cardiac surgery, each launched in 1967: heart transplantation and coronary artery bypass grafting. No prize was awarded for either technique. Why? Consider the case of bypass surgery.[28] It is reasonable to assume that bypass surgery might have been nominated for a prize. The operation provided a successful treatment for coronary artery disease, a disease that was the leading cause of death in Europe and the United States throughout the twentieth century. It is now the leading cause of death worldwide. After the first large case series on bypass surgery was reported in 1968, the procedure quickly caught on. By 1977 US surgeons performed over 100,000 coronary bypass operations each year. The procedure quickly spread around the globe.

Despite its impact on cardiac surgery and on the lives of millions of patients worldwide, bypass surgery has not been recognized with a Nobel Prize. While it is only possible to speculate at this point, there are many reasons why it might have been difficult to award a Nobel for bypass surgery. First, it would be hard to define exactly what innovation the prize would be awarded for – for the idea, for its first clinical use, or for its first success in a large case series? Second, it would be hard to decide which individual should receive the prize.

Most surgeons give most of the credit for bypass surgery to two Cleveland surgeons: Donald Effler and René Favaloro.[29] In 1967 and 1968 they used the procedure in hundreds of patients and convinced their colleagues that it was a viable and valuable approach. But Favaloro simply adapted a technique – saphenous vein grafting – that was already used by vascular surgeons in other parts of the body, for instance to repair renal artery stenosis. Moreover, many other surgeons in the 1950s and 1960s had tried the technique (using either a saphenous vein graft or an internal mammary artery graft) before Favaloro, including Gordon Murray (in animals), Robert Goetz, David Sabiston, Michael DeBakey, and Leningrad surgeon Vasili Kollesov.[30] Consider the case of DeBakey, then the most famous surgeon in the United States, who led a large team of surgeons to develop new techniques of vascular surgery. His team tested coronary bypass surgery in dogs in the early 1960s, but they could not get the technique to work reliably. The grafts, for instance, often did not remain patent

---

28   Jones 2017.
29   Captur 2004; Favaloro 1998.
30   Jones 2013; Jones 2017; Mueller, Todd, Rosengart et al. 1997.

several months after the operation. DeBakey focused his clinical effort on a different technique, coronary endarterectomy. In one operation in November 1964, he and Edward Garret ran into trouble: their attempt to remove the plaque damaged the coronary artery beyond repair. Faced with this emergency, Garret and DeBakey performed a saphenous vein bypass from the aorta. The patient survived the procedure but experienced a peri-operative infarction. They did not attempt another bypass until after Favaloro's report and they did not publish their 1964 case until 1973.[31]

Even though recent nominations are not yet available in the Nobel Archive, we know from other sources that DeBakey was nominated for his work on open heart surgery by Joseph Murray in 2003 (again, surgeons tend to nominate surgeons). The nomination emphasized DeBakey's many contributions to open-heart surgery, as well as his work in medical diplomacy:

> Open-heart surgery has been a major contribution to the treatment of patients world-wide in the past half-century. Its import has not yet been recognized by the Nobel Foundation... One of the greatest achievements of the 20th century was the development of cardio-pulmonary bypass surgery by Michael DeBakey ... Dr. DeBakey has earned a worldwide reputation as an international medical statesman and humanitarian. He has served as advisor to almost every President of the United States over the past fifty years and to heads-of-state throughout the world. ...He often took his team to perform and demonstrate cardiovascular operative procedures, while training his foreign colleagues throughout the globe. For his pioneering contributions to medicine and to humanity, Dr. DeBakey is nominated for the 2003 Nobel Prize in Medicine or Physiology [sic].[32]

This brief review demonstrates a few important points. First, the idea of bypass surgery itself was widespread in the 1960s. Whether the idea had occurred independently to many surgeons, had spread from one surgeon to another, or had been adapted from techniques already in use by surgeons operating on other parts of the body, there were many people who had the idea of using a graft of some sort to restore blood flow to the coronary arteries. Second, many people who did early procedures either did not publish their results (DeBakey and Sabiston), or published them in a way that obscured (Goetz) or undermined (Kolessov, whose article was accompanied by a critical commentary from the

---

31   Garrett, Dennis, DeBakey 1973.
32   Countway Library, HMSc113, Box 55, Folder 28 (DeBakey, Michael, Nobel nomination).

journal editor and from Effler) their accomplishment.[33] While Favaloro was clearly not the first person to perform coronary artery bypass, it was his work that convinced many other surgeons that the technique was viable and worth developing. Favaloro can thus claim the credit for having converted an idea into a major procedure.

Why was the idea so widespread? It may simply have been intuitively obvious to surgeons in Cleveland, New York, Leningrad, Baltimore, and Houston. It is also possible that there was a common ancestor of all of these ideas. The earliest account that we have found of bypass surgery is provided by none other than Alexis Carrel. Carrel described his attempt to use a segment of carotid artery to bypass the proximal coronary artery in a dog in 1910.[34] However, he could not make the procedure work: the surgery took him five minutes, but the dog went into ventricular fibrillation after just three minutes and died. He speculated that it might be possible to perform the technique more quickly, using a Payr ring, which was exactly the technique that Goetz utilized fifty years later. So perhaps no prize was awarded for bypass surgery in the 1960s and 1970s because the committee concluded that the prize-worthy aspect of the innovation had already been awarded to Carrel.

As in many Nobel-worthy innovations, it is difficult to determine whether credit should go to the person who developed the idea, the person who first performed the operation on a patient, or the person who developed the procedure into a large clinical program. Perhaps the committee feared getting drawn into a priority fight between the US and USSR at the height of the Cold War. It could also be that they did not see the procedure as important enough, either because it was only US surgeons who were thoroughly enthusiastic about the procedure, or because it was quickly over-shadowed by coronary angioplasty – a technique that likely produced its own Nobel nominations. It is also possible that the committee saw bypass surgery as a trivial adaptation of Carrel's work, in which case the rise of bypass surgery in the 1960s simply demonstrated the value of the committee's 1912 decision. We look forward to seeing what secrets the archives reveal when they are made accessible for historical research.

Neurosurgery and Brain Surgery

Like transplant and cardiac surgery, brain surgery was also seen as a spectacular transgression of the traditional limits of surgical work and a triumph

---

33   Konstantinov and Goetz 2000; Konstantinov and Kolesov 2004.
34   Carrel 1910.

of twentieth century surgical achievement. A selection of nominations and evaluations show that some neurosurgeons were in principle good candidates for the Nobel Prize. Like all Nobel laureates, Alexis Carrel was invited to nominate scholars for the award each year. In 1932, Carrel chose Harvey Cushing as candidate:

> It seems to me that the contributions made by Harvey Cushing to neurological surgery through the development of his admirable technique, to the anatomical knowledge of the tumors of the brain, and to the physiology of the hypophysis are analogue to those made by Theodor Kocher to the surgery of the thyroid gland many years ago, and for which the Nobel Prize was awarded to him.[35]

Cushing was neither the first nor the last nominee in the field. During the first decade of the Prize, Alfred London put forward Victor Horsley (who later, in 1913, also was nominated by Theodor Kocher),[36] and still during the 1950's, scholars like Wilder Penfield and John Farquhar Fulton were proposed. According to the Nobel committee evaluator in 1954, Fulton's work had links to Moniz' research recognized with the Prize in 1949. Thus, it would be impossible to hand it to him 'post festum'.[37]

Victor Horsley, Harvey Cushing, and Wilder Penfield ended up on different shortlists of the Nobel Committee in various years.[38] However, although both Horsley and Cushing were viewed as prize-worthy by some individuals in the prize jury, only António Egas Moniz was eventually awarded the prize in 1949 for the introduction of frontal lobotomy, an intervention that would no longer be prize-worthy from today's perspective. Moniz had been nominated by 18 scientists from 1928 to 1950 for two achievements: cerebral angiography and lobotomy.[39] In 1936, Moniz published a monograph which described the operation of prefrontal lobotomy and the impressive results of its application to twenty cases of psychosis. At first, lobotomy received mixed reports from some reviewers, because it was mutilating and the negative side effects were still unclear. However, in the Nobel evaluation written in 1949, it was argued

---

35   Alexis Carrel, Yearbook 1932.
36   Yearbook 1910; 'I beg to suggest Sir Victor Horsley, of London, for the Nobel Prize, on account of his distinguished work in connection with the Brain & Cord, & also in connection with the Thyroid gland. I am, Gentlemen, Your obedient Servant, Alfred London, M.D.' Yearbook 1910 (Nobel Archive).
37   Yearbook 1954 (Nobel Archive).
38   Hansson and Schlich 2015b.
39   Stolt 2002.

that lobotomy was 'a great therapeutic step forward'.[40] At that time lobotomy was already acknowledged in some countries. In 1949 about 5,000 lobotomies had been performed in the United States alone. The choice of the Nobel Assembly was discussed in *Nature*, where it was positively acclaimed that Moniz had exerted an important influence, because he directed the attention of neuro-surgeons to psychiatric problems, and revived 'in psychiatry a tradition of courageous and energetic treatment, and he demonstrated that skillful intervention may yield a degree of success even in the most serious and advanced cases of psychosis'.[41]

We could not find much information in the nominations that mentioned patients who had benefitted from the innovations in question. One exception was the highlighted boldness of brain surgeons, leading to discussions concerning patient risk. In 1909, the Nobel Prize reviewer Frithiof Lennmalm suggested that Horsley 'dares to perform bold new interventions on the brain. However, even if he has a breathtaking experimental skill, he sometimes thinks more like an experimental physiologist than as a reflective clinician'.[42] This insinuation of recklessness indirectly pointed to a Horsley's possible indifference towards the patient as the potential victim of such boldness. The role of the patient was later brought up again in the Nobel nominations of Wilder Penfield. Besides describing how Penfield's work that had 'made possible the mapping of a part of the human cortex and should open a new chapter in the physiology of the brain',[43] his nominators, here Albert Bertrand, stressed his patient-centered care:

> Dr. Penfield has organized controlled clinical observation of the physiology and patho-physiology of the human brain to an extent not hitherto achieved, using techniques of stimulation and excision. These techniques were always applied for the benefit of the patient, not simply for experiment. From these operations have come outstanding contributions to the problems of focal epilepsy, cerebral sensory and motor elaboration and the localization of memory patterns and sensory perception. [...] Respectfully yours, W.R. Ingram.[44]

Cushing, with around 40 nominations but no prize, therefore falls into a category of what historian Franz Luttenberger provocatively has called 'highly

---

40   Stolt 2002.
41   Hansson and Schlich 2015.
42   Yearbook 1909 (Nobel Archive).
43   Yearbook 1958 (Nobel Archive).
44   Yearbook 1954 (Nobel Archive).

qualified losers'.[45] His sponsors portrayed Cushing as 'the world's greatest cerebral surgeon'.[46] Many stressed his contributions to the field of brain surgery in general and operations on intracranial tumors in particular, especially in terms of the decreased operation mortality rate. In 1931, the Swedish neurologist Henry Marcus wrote in his evaluation that Cushing had managed to decrease the operative mortality rate to 10% by using x-rays to diagnose brain tumors, electrical stimuli to study of the human sensory cortex, and the electrocautery tool to achieve optimal hemostasis. Therefore, Marcus wrote, such operations were not a 'danse macabre' any longer.[47] The last Nobel committee evaluation on Cushing was written by the neurologist Nils Antoni in 1936. According to Antoni, Cushing had contributed with numerous 'mosaic stones' to the field of brain surgery. Taken together, they had brought about groundbreaking results. The total value of all these contributions would justify a Prize. Another nominator, Friedrich von Müller, even wrote that Cushing had 'become the teacher of all surgeons of the world'.[48] But such a compliment is too general. It is not what Nobel Prizes are awarded for. Compared to the Moniz' nominations, Cushing's nominators did not pinpoint one major achievement. To the contrary, the nominators provided detailed explanations of various accomplishments. In this way, they eluded the 'breakthrough' model.

Conclusion

Historians and sociologists have long been interested in the role of excellence, credit and priority in medicine. Case studies of Nobel Prize nominations and Nobel committee reports offer important contributions to this discussion. As Robert Friedman has pointed out, winning a Nobel Prize has never been an automatic process.[49] We believe it is important to look into how excellence has been attributed in order to deepen our understanding of reward mechanisms in medicine. In our case study of nominated (or possibly nominated) transplant, cardiac, and brain surgeons, we have found an emphasis on ideas of genius, scientific heroism, boldness, as well as utopian visions of the scientific solution of seemingly insurmountable problems.

---

45   Luttenberger 1996.
46   Hansson and Schlich 2015.
47   Yearbook 1931 (Nobel Archive).
48   Hansson, Schlich 2015.
49   Friedman 2001.

In the discussions at the various levels of the prize awarding procedure one can see certain patterns. It is clearly not enough to be an excellent surgeon, not even to be 'the best surgeon in the world', 'the teacher of all surgeons in the world', or the researcher behind an eponym, may it be Cushing's disease, Murphy's button, or the Blalock-Taussig-shunt. Judging by the four individuals who have been awarded the Nobel Prize for the development of surgical procedures, excellence was measured by the potential impact of a particular discovery or innovation, especially when that innovation opened up a new area of surgical work. The construction of devices (like the heart-lung-machine), whether used in surgery or not, have also mostly not convinced the Nobel jury (the exception that proves the rule is Willem Einthoven's Nobel Prize in 1924 'for his discovery of the mechanism of the electrocardiogram'). The same is true for mere technical improvements or a contribution to an ongoing development in the field. Similarly, a broad range of achievements, or gradual successful work was also not a route to a Nobel Prize. Instead, nominators had to highlight a 'breakthrough' discovery or innovation that had broad consequences. In addition, it had to be a breakthrough that could clearly be attributed to one, two or three individual scientists. Surgery offered a unique way of impressing the committee with innovations that went beyond the traditional limits of medical possibilities or even broke 'taboos'. Transplant, brain, and heart surgery all fit that mold. But that is a very narrow way of defining excellence, one that fits surgery only in a few specific cases. It includes Moniz, whom we would no longer reward with a Nobel Prize, but not Cushing, Penfield, Blalock and Taussig, all of whom remain prize-worthy in the eyes of modern surgeons. They embody an excellence that is more typical for surgery today. It may be that surgical excellence, as generally understood does not align well with the excellence that is normally recognized with a Nobel Prize.

As mentioned before, the question for us is not so much whether the decisions of the Nobel Committee were the right or the wrong ones, or whether a given surgeon's achievements ought to have been impressive enough to win the prize. Instead, it is more a question of what kind of achievement was considered the most important and the most excellent at a particular time. There is no way to objectively measure such a thing. It is not a question of the presence or absence of excellence, or of 'how much' excellence there was. Instead, it was a question of the nature of excellence. The decision-making process and the award of the Prize itself is an example of enacting excellence, in the sense that we look at excellence as being dependent of its acknowledgment and attribution. Excellence as a category for surgery comes into being by being determined and performed in that process. Seen that way, awarding the 'crown jewel of excellence' to António Egas Moniz, for example, was not 'wrong', it was how excellence at that point in time was enacted through the Nobel Prize mechanism.

Acknowledgments

Files on surgeons in the Nobel archive were kindly provided by the Nobel Committee for Physiology or Medicine. Translations from Swedish, German and French into English were made by the authors.

Bibliography

Blatchford, J.W. and Rehn, L. 1985. 'The First Successful Cardiography'. *Annals of Thoracic Surgery* 39: 492–495.

Captur, G. 2004. 'Memento for René Favaloro'. *Texas Heart Institute Journal* 31: 47–60.

Carrel, A. 1910. 'On the Experimental Therapy of the Thoracic Aorta and the Heart'. *Annals of Surgery* 52: 83–95.

Crawford, E. (ed.). 2002. *Historical Studies in the Nobel Archives: The Prizes in Science and Medicine*. Tokyo: Universal Academy Press.

Duffin, J. 2010. *History of Medicine, A Scandalously Short Introduction*. Toronto: University of Toronto Press.

Favaloro, G.R. 1998. 'Landmarks in the Development of Coronary Artery Bypass Surgery'. *Circulation* 98: 466–478.

Frampton, S. 2016. 'Honour and subsistence: invention, credit and surgery in the nineteenth century'. *British Journal for the History of Science* 49 (4): 561–576.

Friedman, R.M. 2001. *The Politics of Excellence: Behind the Nobel Prize in Science*. New York: Times Books.

Garrett, H.E.; Dennis, E.W.; DeBakey, M.E. 1973. 'Aortocoronary Bypass with Saphenous Vein Graft: Seven-Year Follow-Up'. *Journal of the American Medical Association* 223: 792–794.

Hansson N., 2015. 'Ein Umschwung des medizinischen Denkens oder eine übereifrige literarische Tätigkeit? August Bier, die Homöopathie und der Nobelpreis 1906–1936'. *Jahrbuch für Medizin, Gesellschaft, Geschichte* 33: 217–246.

Hansson, N. and Schlich, T. 2015a. 'Why did Alfred Blalock and Helen Taussig not receive the Nobel Prize?'. *Journal of Cardiac Surgery* 30: 506–509.

Hansson, N. and Schlich, T. 2015b. 'Highly qualified loser? Harvey Cushing and the Nobel Prize'. *Journal of Neurosurgery* 122: 976–979.

Hansson, N.; Fangerau, H.; Tuffs, A. et al. 2016. 'No Silver Medal for Nobel Prize Contenders: Why Anesthesia Pioneers Were Nominated for but Denied the Award'. *Anesthesiology* 125 (1): 34–38.

Hansson, N; Halling, T; Fangerau, H. 2016. 'The Nobel Prize and Otolaryngology: Papa Gunnar's promotion of his peers Gustav Killian and Themistocles Gluck'. *Acta Oto-Laryngologica* 136 (9): 871–874.

Hansson, N.; Halling, T.; Moll, F. et al. 2017. 'Berühmte Gynäkologen. Deutsche Nobelpreiskandidaten in der Gynäkologie 1901–1920'. *Geburtshilfe Frauenheilkunde*. Stuttgart and New York: Georg Thieme Verlag KG.

Hansson, N. 2018. Excellence in orthopaedic surgery: an overview of Nobel Prize nominees 1901–1960 with focus on Friedrich Pauwels and Gerhard Küntscher. *International Orthopaedics* 42 (12): 2957–2960.

Jones, D.S. 2013. *Broken Hearts: The Tangled History of Cardiac Care*. Baltimore: Johns Hopkins University Press.

Jones, D.S. 2017. 'Surgical Practice and the Reconstruction of the Therapeutic Niche: The Case of Myocardial Revascularization'. In *Technological Change in Modern Surgery: Historical Perspectives on Innovation*, edited by T. Schlich and C. Crenner, 185–216. Rochester: University of Rochester Press.

Jordanova, L. 1995. 'The social construction of medical knowledge'. *Social History of Medicine* 8 (3): 361–381.

Konstantinov, I.E. and Goetz, R.H. 2000. 'The Surgeon Who Performed the First Successful Clinical Coronary Artery Bypass Operation'. *Annals of Thoracic Surgery* 69: 1966–1972.

Konstantinov, I.E. and Kolesov, V.I. 2004. 'A Surgeon to Remember'. *Texas Heart Institute Journal* 31: 349–358.

Lawrence, C. 1992. 'Democratic, Divine and Heroic: The History and Historiography of Surgery'. In *Medical Theory and Surgical Practice: Studies in the History of Surgery*, edited by Christopher Lawrence, 1–47. London: Routledge.

Le Vay, D. and Carrel, A. 1996. *The Perfectibility of Man*. Rockville: Kabel Publishing.

Luttenberger, F. 1996. 'Excellence and chance: the Nobel Prize case of E. von Behring and É. Roux'. *History and Philosophy of the Life Sciences* 18: 225–238.

Monagan, D. and Williams, D.O. 2007. *Journey into the Heart: A Tale of Pioneering Doctors and Their Race to Transform Cardiovascular Medicine*. New York: Gotham Books.

Moore, F.D. 1995. *A Miracle and a Privilege. Recounting a Half Century of Surgical Advance*. Washington, D.C.: National Academy Press.

Mueller, R.L.; Todd, K.; Rosengart, T.K. et al. 1997. 'The History of Surgery for Ischemic Heart Disease'. *Annals of Thoracic Surgery* 63: 869–878.

Murray, J.E. 2001. *Surgery of the Soul. Reflections on a Curious Career*. Boston: Boston Medical Library/Science History Publications/USA.

Reverby, S. and Rosner, D. 2004. 'Beyond the Great Doctors' Revisited. A Generation of the New Social History of Medicine'. In *Locating Medical History. The Stories and Their Meaning*, edited by F. Huisman and J. Harley Warner, 167–193. Baltimore and London: JHU Press.

Schlich, T. 2007. 'Nobel Prizes for Surgeons: In Recognition of the Surgical Healing Strategy.' *International Journal of Surgery* (5): 129–133.

Schlich, T. 2010. *The Origins of Organ Transplantation: Surgery and Laboratory Science, 1880s–1930s.* Rochester and New York: The University of Rochester Press.

Schlich, T. 2016. 'One and the Same the World Over: The International Culture of Surgical Exchange'. *Journal of the History of Medicine and Allied Sciences* 71 (3): 247–270.

Stolt, C.M. 2002. 'Moniz, lobotomy, and the 1949 Nobel Prize'. In *Historical Studies in the Nobel Archives: The Prizes in Science and Medicine,* edited by E.T. Crawford, 79–94. Tokyo: Universal Academy Press.

Tröhler, U. 1984. *Auf dem Weg zur physiologischen Chirurgie. Der Nobelpreisträger Theodor Kocher 1841–1917.* Basel, Boston and Stuttgart: Birkhäuser.

Tröhler, U. 2013. 'Theodor Kochers Nobelpreis: Voraussetzungen, Bedingungen, Folgen. Ein Blick hinter die Kulissen'. In *Schnitten, Knoten und Netze. 100 Jahre schweizerische Gesellschaft für Chirurgie,* edited by H. Steinke; E. Wolff and R.A. Schmid, 87–110. Zürich: Chronos Verlag.

Woolgar, S.W. 1976. 'Writing an Intellectual History of Scientific Development: The Use of Discovery Accounts'. *Social Studies of Science* 6: 395–422.

Zuckerman, H. 1977. *Scientific Elite. Nobel Laureates in the United States.* London: MacMillan.

PART 3

Reverberation and Commercialization

∵

John C. Eccles' Conversion and the Meaning of 'Authority'

Fabio De Sio, Nils Hansson and Ulrich Koppitz

Robert K. Merton's tentative taxonomy of the 'instructively ambiguous' categories of 'excellence' and 'recognition' features the Nobel Prize as an example of the couple 'excellence as performance/recognition as honorific'.[1] In this connection, Merton raises the problem of what the performance to be recognised should look like. In the sciences, he concludes, the single achievement (as opposed to 'life-work'[2]) seems to be the standard, although what this means is far from self-evident.

Alfred Nobel's three famous criteria for a prize-worthy achievement ('recency', 'benefit to mankind' and 'discovery') have equally proven difficult to handle, requiring progressive adjustments (see the Introduction to this volume). In situations of real-life complexity, Merton's taxonomy of 'recognition' and 'excellence as performance' shows its analytical limit, as do Nobel's criteria. Even in early, apparently simple, cases of undivided awards, the stumbling block of the 'individual discovery' had made itself perspicuous, as shown by the lengthy debate over Ivan Pavlov's[3] or Paul Ehrlich's award,[4] demonstrating how problematic the 'snapshot' conception of discovery can be. One is here reminded of Roland Barthes' concept of 'punctum',[5] '[the] element which rises from the scene, shoots out of it like an arrow, and pierces [us]'. The 'punctum' is what commands our attention and makes us notice an image. This event, however, can only be perceived as such within the less perspicuous framework of an educated and idiosyncratic approach, which he calls 'studium', and is the 'application to a thing [...] a kind of general, enthusiastic commitment, but without special acuity'.[6] Transposed to the problem at hand, the 'punctum' can be abruptly translated as '(beneficial) discovery', whereas 'studium' becomes the set of conditions that makes the achievement recognised as a great

---

1 Merton 1973.
2 Merton 1973, 433.
3 Todes 2002, Chapter 10.
4 Hüntelmann 2018.
5 Barthes 1981, 26.
6 Barthes 1981, 26.

contribution to a specific field. Since it provides the background for our punctual awareness of the event, the 'studium' requires some effort to be acknowledged at all.

In what follows, we will attempt the analysis of one famous Nobel laureate from a perspective complementary to that of the binomial excellence/recognition, namely, that of 'authority'. Although no less ambiguous than the couple it is intended to replace, the concept we propose is just as productive: it allows to consider the co-evolution of discovery[7] (individual level) and honorific recognition (community), their articulation, the process of maturation of both the knowledge claims and technical innovations that are considered 'discoveries', and the general and local criteria that sanction them as such. In other words, we will try in this case to show the inevitable interdependence of 'punctum' and 'studium'.

The case is the 1963 award given to the Australian physiologist John C. Eccles (1903–1997), with Alan L. Hodgkin and Andrew F. Huxley, 'for their discoveries concerning the ionic mechanisms involved in excitation and inhibition in the peripheral and central portions of the nerve cell membrane'. The focus will be on Eccles, the first in the official list of the awardees, a towering figure in the history of neurophysiology and the neurosciences.[8]

Conversion and the Creation of Authority

Eccles' scientific upbringing took place between 1927 and 1937, in a Mecca of physiological science, the Oxford laboratory of Charles Scott Sherrington, where he directly participated in the completion and refinement of his master's life-work on spinal reflexes, rewarded with a Nobel Prize in 1932. In the eyes of his pupil, the old 'figurehead' of British science[9] was an authority in every sense, a model he tried to follow and match, also beyond the laboratory walls. Eccles borrowed the master's experimental approach, integrative outlook,[10] and focus on inhibition as a bona fide physiological mechanism.[11]

---

7   Throughout the present chapter, we will use 'discovery' as a synonym of 'excellence as performance' in Merton's sense.

8   Curtis and Andersen 2001.

9   Smith 2000; see also Smith 1992; Smith 2001; Smith 2003.

10   on which see Sherrington 1906.

11   On the debate over the statute of inhibition (mechanism vs. simple physical consequence of the refractory period after discharge) see Granit 1961, Chapter IV; Jacobson 1993, Chapter 4; Smith 1992, Chapter 5.

Not least, he fashioned himself as an apostle of Sherrington's Cartesian-dualistic view of man.[12]

As a consequence of his collaboration with Sherrington, in a series of studies on the summation of impulses at the synapse in the early 1930s, Eccles became involved[13] in one of the harshest controversies in the history of neurophysiology: the dispute over the nature (chemical or electrical) of synaptic transmission, aka 'the war of the soups and the sparks'.[14] The hypothesis, championed since the 1910s by some pharmacologists, that acetylcholine played a central role in the transmission of the nerve impulse at every level (neuromyal junction and spinal neurones) had met fierce resistance from 'proper' neurophysiologists, who favoured a physical (electrical) interpretation in analogy with the mechanism of conduction along the axon.

Eccles quickly rose to the leadership of the electrical side. His knowledge of the physiology of reflexes, experimental ingenuity and pugnacity made him, in the words of a witness, 'the one to whom all the non-believers made reference when they had run out of arguments'.[15] He approached the problem at the level of the neuromuscular junction, sensory ganglia and motor cells, piling a mountain of evidence against a hypothesis which he considered insufficient to account for the essential quantitative details (speed, summative character) of synaptic transmission. The main theatre of the dispute were the meetings of the Physiological Society, where he staged memorable fights with the leading 'chemagonist'[16] and future Nobel laureate (1936) Henry H. Dale and associates, often to the embarrassment of the session chairs. The personal relations among the fighters, however, and especially those between Eccles and Dale, were not in the least harmed, as is testified by the eyewitness Bernhard Katz (1996) and the correspondence among the protagonists (fraught with military metaphors).[17] Dale and his group privately and publicly acknowledged the beneficial effect of Eccles' criticism (forcing them to refine experimentation and theory to meet the standards of the neurophysiologists), as well as the balance and measure he displayed in the occasional role of the reviewer.[18]

---

12   Sherrington 1938; but see on this Smith 2000; De Sio 2018.

13   Curtis and Andersen 2001.

14   Valenstein 2002; Valenstein 2006.

15   Bacq 1974, 62; For a full history of the controversy see Valenstein 2006; Shepherd 2009; Bennett 2001; Borck 2017.

16   'Chemagonists' was the collective name coined by Walter Cannon (1939) for the supporters of chemical transmission. Their opponents he called 'electragonists'.

17   Partly published in Eccles 1976; Eccles 1982; Girolami et al. 1994; two letters also in Freund et al. 2011.

18   See Dale to Eccles 29/1/37, Eccles Archives, Medizingeschichte Düsseldorf (EAMD) 2NZ-2023.

Nevertheless, Eccles' 'super aggressive personality'[19] did not fit the Oxonian style and raised more than an eyebrow. When Sherrington retired in 1936, his pupil's aspirations to succession were thwarted, leaving him no choice but to accept a research position in his native Australia. The rest of the story has been recounted several times by the protagonist,[20] echoed by pupils and hagiographers, finally making its way into historiography. It is a story of endless meandering (from Sydney to Dunedin, New Zealand and back to Canberra), isolation, and frustration, but also of great achievement against all odds, of an astonishing inversion of the centre-periphery power relations in wartime, and of a mighty new school of neurophysiology being born down under.[21] Most perspicuously, however, it is a story of conversions.

At a most delicate juncture in his career, as the electrical theory of synaptic transmission was progressively buried under a snowfall of contrary evidence,[22] Eccles came under the spell of the philosopher Karl Popper. According to his own, oft-repeated account[23] Popper liberated him from the 'inductive dogma', persuading him of the necessity of clear-cut hypotheses, and that falsification of one's own theories is not a shame. With his guidance, Eccles set to work to formulate a theoretical version of his electrical hypotheses of synaptic excitation[24] and inhibition,[25] with predictions and possible tests, and then tried to disprove them. The inhibition theory was the first to fall under the fire 'of his own Popperian architect',[26] in a fateful summer night of 1951. The model was based on the competition between the sensory stimuli (excitatory), and the interfering action of some short-axon interneurones, the 'Golgi cells', which, once activated by collaterals of afferent axons, subliminally depolarized the motoneurone, making it inert to the following trains of impulses from the receptors. Critical to the testing of this hypothesis was a technical novelty, intracellular electrodes – electrical probes with a tip so fine that it could be inserted into a vertebrate neurone, allowing direct measurement of its activity. Eccles chose to 'impale' the large and relatively well-known spinal motoneurones innervating the quadriceps muscle of the cat's thigh, the so-called 'monosynaptic pathway', characterised by David P. Lloyd in the 1940s. The electrical hypothesis predicted a depolarisation the membrane, making the internal electrode

---

19   Shepherd 2009, 74.
20   Eccles 1966; Eccles 1970; Eccles 1977.
21   On which, see Stuart and Pierce 2006.
22   Bennett 2001.
23   Eccles 1966; Eccles 1970; Eccles 1975; Eccles 1982.
24   Eccles 1945; Eccles 1946.
25   Brooks and Eccles 1947.
26   Shepherd 2009, 93.

record a positive potential. If, on the contrary, the inhibition was chemical, then the recorded potential was expected to be negative due to hyperpolarisation.[27] The signal on the cathode-ray amplifier went down – the electrical theory was 'thereby falsified'.[28] One month later Eccles left for a long trip to the US and UK, carrying the news of his 'belated conversion'[29] – consequence of the philosophical one seven years before. Many neurophysiologists were taken aback, but the pharmacologists feasted on it privately and publicly. In a 1953 meeting, Dale compared Eccles to St. Paul on the way to Damascus, when 'the scales fell from his eyes'.[30] On that occasion, the pharmacologist F.H. Shaw went on to draw the necessary consequences: 'In view of Eccles abandonment of electrical transmission [...] it can be said with some certainty that transmission in the [sensory] ganglion is [also] humoral'.[31]

With this sudden move, General Eccles managed to successfully change sides without losing his grades. In this case, authority and conversion stand in a relation of simultaneous contrast, mutually enhancing their respective intensity. Since 'such a high voltage spark as Eccles'[32] had espoused the chemical theory, then it had to be not only true, but also universal. On the other hand, having 'kill[ed] his own brainchild',[33] and so effectively, made him not only a leader of the chemical side, but also a champion of proper scientific method.

Historiographical accounts of this event have been informed by this philosophical outlook, deducing the change in epistemic strategy from the epistemological conversion, and consequently magnifying the import of the 'crucial experiment'. A participant observer like Bacq[34] casts the end of the 'war' as early as 1945, the year Eccles met Popper. Others set it in 1952,[35] the year the experiment was published.[36] To Bennett 'so concluded the long saga that

---

27 For details, see Eccles 1957.

28 Brock et al. 1952; see also Eccles 1982.

29 Eccles 1982, 334.

30 Dale 1954.

31 Shaw 1954. To which statement Archibald McIntyre (Eccles' former associate and his successor in Dunedin) replied abruptly: '[...] the sudden rejection of his former creed by an old and formidable electrical antagonist seems to some a sufficient substitute for positive and substantial proof [...] I cannot see how Eccles' views on central synapses should in any way affect one's thinking about ganglia. If there is a case for chemical transmission in ganglia, surely it rests on its own feet' (McIntyre 1954).

32 McIntyre 1954.

33 Eccles 1966.

34 Bacq 1974.

35 Valenstein 2002; Valenstein 2006; Shepherd 2008; Shepherd 2009; Dupont 1999.

36 Brock et al. 1952. From a more nuanced perspective, Robinson (2001) dates the end of the controversy in 1965.

established the supremacy of chemical transmission',[37] or, in the even more emphatic words of an occasional historian: 'Chief Spark had capitulated. The battle was over'.[38] Following Eccles' own lead, the 1951 microelectrode trials were made into an 'eureka' experience, which, 'at a stroke, falsified the theory of electrical transmission',[39] or, in a most un-Popperian interpretation, they became 'the experiment that proved chemical transmission'.[40]

This 'punctum' (the juxtaposition of epistemological-cum-epistemic change and crucial experiment), so forcefully catching the eye of retrospective observers, is not in itself deceiving. Yet, it can engender optical (intellectual) illusions, if we do not consider the underlying 'studium'. An assessment of the historical meaning of Eccles' work to neurophysiology, we argue, is better served by shifting the focus from the question of truth (what this one experiment demonstrated) to that of productivity (what the renovated experimental system allowed). From this perspective, Borck has compellingly shown that Eccles' conversion to falsificationism has always remained at best partial; that the 'integra[tion of] innovative methods', often contributed by collaborators[41] was of greater importance than his 'novel philosophical approach'; and that the 'crucial experiment'[42] had not determined, but at best sanctioned the demise of the electrical dead horse. All of which leads us to the issue of conversion. There is no ground for contending that, subjectively, there was no such moment. What matters is rather how this happened, how Eccles had seen it coming, how he had already progressively adjusted his views[43] and, finally, how he had found in the Popperian method a second chance he was quick to seize.[44] In 1951, Borck argues, our hero 'was ready to give up on electrical transmission [...], as his experimental system was flying on autopilot by then'.[45]

Rather than by the disproof of a particular wrong hypothesis, the decisive change was brought by the coming of age of Eccles' own 'machine for making the future',[46] just as good for generating questions as it was for providing answers, in an endless resonance among different levels (theory; models;

---

37   Bennett 2001, 38.
38   Gross 2013.
39   Fillenz 2000; see also Fillenz 2012.
40   Todman 2008; see also Karczmar 2001.
41   Borck 2017, 323.
42   The 'crucial experiment' is more realistically cast as the culmination of a series of carefully planned trials started in the spring of 1951. See also Stuart and Brownstone 2011.
43   See the example provided by Bacq 1974; see also Eccles 1946, 448.
44   Dupont (1999) nastily calls the Popperian conversion a 'philosophical alibi'.
45   Borck 2017, 325.
46   Rheinberger 1997, 28.

observation; technique; disciplines; institutions). In the decade between Eccles' conversion and his Nobelisation, the system consolidated itself progressively, if not linearly, with new perspectives opened by theoretical necessities, the input of new recruits and even technical challenges. The motoneurones of the monosynaptic pathway were turned by Eccles not only into the test ground of the theory, but into a candidate model-system for synaptology.[47] To this end, the basic physiological measures (the potentials) were incorporated in a simplified theoretical neurone[48] and the membrane was singled out as the really active element that, through its selective porosity to different ions, made the game of excitation and inhibition possible.[49] The focus on the membrane (rather than the whole cell) was at once a simplifying element of the system, and a point of connection with distant research programmes, such as that of the biophysicist Alan Hodgkin and the Cambridge axonologists (especially Andrew F. Huxley), a rapprochement with which Eccles had long sought.[50] The microelectrodes provided the means for such a dialogue,[51] allowing him to match, in whole-animal, complex system, the degree of precision and control afforded by the isolated squid-axon preparations used at Cambridge. A decisive step forward in this direction was marked by turning an experimental complication (the fact that the glass microelectrodes leaked some of the saline solution they contained) into an asset: the development of a double-barrelled microelectrode capable of electrophoretically injecting ions in the neurone, while at the same time measuring the potential changes.[52] These technical, theoretical and disciplinary displacements (his laboratory had to expand its activity to neuropharmacology and neuroanatomy), provided in turn the elements of Eccles' system of neurophysiology.[53] Also the anatomical and physiological details of the model underwent much transformation. Interneurones, initially part of the electrical theory of inhibition (the 'Golgi cells') and thus falsified, re-appeared in 1952–55 thanks to the input of Paul Fatt, this time in

---

47   Eccles 1953.

48   A sphere with 7 cylindrical dendrites, Eccles 1952; Eccles 1953; Coombs et al. 1955; Coombs et al. 1959.

49   Fillenz 2011; Curtis and Andersen 2001.

50   The occasional but never casual correspondence between the two (preserved in EAMD/2NZ-2051 and /2AU2063) amply testifies to this.

51   Eccles' appropriation of Hodgkin's model of the membrane as an electrical resistance and acceptance of the 'sodium pump' hypothesis further facilitated the dialogue. See Eccles 1953.

52   Although Eccles (1957) proposes this interpretation of such fundamental development, Shepherd 2008; Shepherd 2009; as well as Stuart and Brownstone (2011) tell a less linear story of appropriation, at the expense of Archibald McIntyre.

53   Eccles 1953.

the form of 'Renshaw cells',[54] and were given a central position in the model. The interneurone hypothesis concurred to the demise of Lloyd's theory of 'direct inhibition'; to the confirmation of 'Dale's Principle',[55] according to which one neurone secretes only one type of neurotransmitter; and to the simplification of network, now neatly divided into specialized excitatory and inhibitory cells.[56] It goes without saying that none of these elements went uncontested,[57] and a few of them did not stand the test of time.[58]

Within this expanding system, the true nature of synaptic transmission was at best an important detail,[59] also because the microelectrode experiments falsified Eccles' own electrical theory, not the (still widely held) conviction that synaptic transmission is electrical, or mainly so.[60] The air was not as 'suddenly cleared' after the 1951 experiment, as a historian would have it,[61] also because the sharp incompatibility of the two mechanisms was a Popperian trick introduced by Eccles, rather than anyone's real persuasion. Finally, a few historiographers[62] have remarked how the crucial experiment, regardless of whether it proved or disproved of any particular theory, was the first experimental demonstration that inhibition is a physiological process (hyperpolarisation of the membrane), independent from – and interacting with – excitation. The cornerstone of Sherrington's theory had been made visible, and was to provide the horizon for almost Eccles' entire experimental career.

The relevant question, then, is not what the 'conversion' purportedly closed (the 'war'), but what it opened: a decade of staggeringly productive research, and an even longer period of diffusion, refinement and evolution

---

54   Eccles 1987.
55   Eccles 1957.
56   Eccles 1957.
57   See one clear example in Casey 2009.
58   Bennett 1985.
59   Borck 2017.
60   One of the reasons why Eccles found it useful to formulate an explicit theory was that, as he noted early on (Eccles 1937), there actually was no theory for electrical synaptic transmission, but just converging data supporting a widely-held persuasion. Moreover, the conversion made Eccles just as many enemies as friends, starting from a few of his former collaborators. See for instance the furious reaction of Chandler McC. Brooks (co-author of the 1945 inhibition hypothesis) in the discussion following Brock et al. 1953 and again in (Brooks 1958). See note 31 above for the reaction of McIntyre, Eccles' successor in Dunedin. In the USA, Ralph Gerard, Alexander Forbes, Rafael Lorente de Nó and David Lloyd (all Nobel pluri-nominees in the 1950s) remained long unconvinced (see Marcum 2006). Doubts were repeatedly expressed by McCulloch and his group (also at the forefront of microelectrode research), and Hebb (1961).
61   Shepherd 2009, 93.
62   Fillenz 2000; Fillenz 2012; Bennett 2001.

of techniques, data and problems springing from the Southern Hemisphere, which would in due course become the torment and delight of the devil's advocates in Stockholm.

Attributing Authority. The Nobel Committee and Eccles

Eccles' 'converted' research programme put him almost at once in the spotlight of the Nobel committee. In the 10 years between 1952 (year of publication of the first experiment with Brock and Coombs) and his actual awarding, Eccles received about twenty nominations.[63]

The first came in January 1953 from the neurologist Richard Jung, who proposed him together with Paul Hoffmann, 'for their discovery of the principles and mechanisms of the transmission of excitation in the Central Nervous System [hereafter CNS]'. Eccles was credited with the discovery of the 'basic mechanism of synaptic excitation and inhibition of neurones in the CNS' and the extension of Hodgkin's membrane model to the vertebrate neurone. Jung put a special emphasis on the quantitative side of Eccles' achievement, on his success in determining the basic facts about the transmission of the nerve impulse by working on structures and problems that were not his own exclusive province. Eccles' older works on synaptic excitation were also mentioned.

In case of a tripartition of the prize, Jung suggested that Hodgkin be included as well, in order to award all 'the most important discoveries in the field of General Physiology'. Eccles' dossier was handed over to his old Oxford colleague Ragnar Granit, whose final judgement was articulated.[64] Eccles' pre-1951 contributions on excitation were considered not worthy of the prize, despite the undeniable contribution they provided to the overall picture of synaptic transmission.[65] The more recent experiments on inhibition[66] were instead considered of Nobel calibre: despite the technique of intracellular recording not having been developed in Eccles' laboratory, there it was first employed in the vertebrate CNS, making the elements of synaptic transmission measurable.

---

63   These nominations are not registered in the Nobel nomination database online, since it to date only covers the nominations from 1901 to 1953.

64   We were not able to access this review, the essentials of which are however summarised in the following reports, as well as in Norrby 2016, Chapter 2.

65   Yearbook of Nobel Proceedings, 1955. Review Bernhard, pp. 1–3. All the citations of nominations and reviews mentioned below will be shortened to the Name/Date form, reference to the corresponding Yearbook being implicit.

66   Brock et al. 1952.

Nevertheless, these experiences and the resulting generalisation were still too recent and contested to warrant a Nobel Prize.

In 1955 Eccles was proposed (with later Nobel laureate Ulf von Euler) by the physiologist Ernst Gellhorn, who emphasized the methodological value of his work, especially the 'introduction of intracellular electrodes'.[67] The review fell on Carl Gustaf Bernhard, Professor of Physiology at the Karolinska Institute. Drawing substantially from the previous year's review, Bernhard dismissed Eccles' pre-1951 production as not worth considering for a prize, and duly contextualised his use of intracellular electrodes within the history of this technique. He admired the success in recording from spinal motoneurones, but was doubtful of the candidate's primacy in this accomplishment. Bernhard concurred with Granit on the import of the intracellular studies, especially the measurements of the resting and action potential they afforded and the perspectives they opened to the analysis of excitatory and inhibitory mechanisms. As to Eccles' model of inhibition, three issues remained: (1) the anatomical pathways supposedly mediating the phenomenon; (2) the possible measurement artefacts caused by intracellular recording; (3) the unequivocal derivation of inhibition from hyperpolarisation of the membrane. On none of these three points could Bernhard find sufficient consensus within the physiological community. As to the first problem, the 'conversion' experiments of 1951 seemed to have ruled out the action of interneurones, re-introduced in subsequent work (1953–1954).[68] Moreover, Eccles' novel enthusiasm for the chemical hypothesis had failed to convince many 'electragonists', including some of his former collaborators. As to the measurement artefacts, reasons for doubt were to be found in the very work of the candidate and of others. The same held for the exclusive relationship between hyperpolarisation and inhibition. Finally, Bernhard expressed reservations on the status of chemical 'transmitters' in the CNS: a number of publications (also by the reviewer) suggested that acetylcholine functioned rather as a modulator than as a transmitter. Despite Popper, the electrical hypothesis was alive, and firing. Bernhard concluded that a prize was still premature.

In 1958, the physiologist János Szentágothai from Pécs nominated Eccles for his work on central inhibition and excitation. The pharmacologist Franz Theodor von Brücke of Vienna also proposed him 'as second nominee' after Hodgkin, with the same motivation, plus a reference to his work on Renshaw cells.[69] In the light of the quantity of new material and problems, Granit

---

67   Nomination Gellhorn 1955.
68   Bernhard 1955, 7–8; Eccles 1957.
69   We could not access the original texts of the nominations. They are however summarised in the opening of Granit's 1958 review (Review Granit 1958, 1). Moreover, Norrby (2016, 95)

(this year's reviewer) engaged in a wholly new analysis. He took objection to Bernhard's 1955 conclusion about the lack of clarity in the excitation-inhibition story. To him, the crux of the question was more whether Eccles could be considered a 'true blood donor', a protagonist of this complicated scientific plot (involving many actors), than to ascertain the exactness and conclusiveness of his own theories.[70] The review was organised in five sections: physiological characteristics of the membrane in ventral horn cells (motoneurones); internal differences in the spread of the impulse (among axon, cell body and dendrites); membrane potential measurements in excitation and inhibition; artificial alteration of the membrane potential (the double-barrelled microelectrode); tonic and phasic motoneurones.[71] As to the first topic, Granit did not add to his own 1953 review, only stressing the comparability of Eccles' results with those of Hodgkin and Huxley on the squid giant axon and recent confirmations by others, stimulated and inspired by the nominee's results.[72] As for the topology of the spread of the impulse along the neurone, it was judged ground-breaking neurophysiology, although the claim to discovery in this case could not be made by Eccles only, and methodological issues persisted.[73]

To Granit, once again, the excitation/inhibition mechanism was the kernel of Eccles' claim to immortality. Problems of interpretation remained, and perhaps the evidence substantiating the model was not decisive but, Granit stressed, it was the complexity of the experimental situation (recording from whole animals, with limited control of the medium conditions) that stood in the way of an unequivocal solution.[74] No conclusive evidence that acetylcholine was the *immediate* cause of membrane depolarisation in excitation had been adduced, and therefore this part of the system had not 'reached the required degree of clarity required for Nobel-class works'.[75] The case for inhibition was to some extent stronger. Granit doubted that membrane hyperpolarisation was the only explanation for it, but acknowledged that different mechanisms would most likely constitute an exception.[76] He stressed, however, that these objections were not meant to downplay Eccles' achievement: in both

states that 'The nominations of Eccles continued in 1956–58'. We were not able to find them, however.

70   Review Granit 1958, 2.
71   Ibid.
72   Ibid, 3.
73   Ibid.
74   Ibid, 8.
75   Ibid, 8.
76   Ibid, 10–11.

cases, he had succeeded in 'adding clarity and precision to the question'[77] and had inspired others, most often with confirmatory results. In the end, Granit mused, 'It would be an extremely strange procedure to deny the value of great discoveries, which means real progress, just because there are still discoveries' in that area. Ditto for the experiments with double-barrelled microelectrodes, which were saluted as a decisive step forward in bringing whole-animal experiments almost to the same level of control as isolated-organ and single-synapse ones: more was simply not achievable.[78] It was the referee's opinion that Eccles' use of the new method had born 'enough factual material for an experimental build-up'. Eccles was declared prize-worthy for having introduced the intracellular recording technique at the level of the spinal cord and, in terms of 'discoveries', for having proven inhibition to be an active process and having defined the essential features of the nerve impulse. From this viewpoint, his researches constituted a pendant of Hodgkin and Huxley's ones on axonal conduction: the three, taken together, had indeed started a 'whole new physiology'.

In 1959, nominations came from J.H.F. Brotherston, on behalf of the Edinburgh Medical Faculty, David Whitteridge (Physiology, Edinburgh) and Peter Bishop (Physiology, Sydney). The collective statement stressed the intrinsic difficulty of Eccles's experiments, as well as the elegant simplicity of the theoretical framework. It also credited him with having done 'much to reconcile the quantitative evidence on the electrical processes' of nerve function in the CNS, with 'ideas of chemical transmission as fertile, but hitherto expressed in less rigorous terms'.[79] Finally, Eccles' long association with Sherrington was mentioned, together with the nerve-muscle work with Katz and Kuffler.[80]

Whitteridge's nomination was a facsimile of Brotherston's, but added Hodgkin as a candidate co-recipient for his 'discovery' of the sodium-mechanism of membrane excitation. 'His work on the isolated axon', Whitteridge commented,

> although more restricted than that of Eccles, is more fundamental and therefore susceptible to a more rigorous experimental approach. Indeed, it has provided the [...] framework for the interpretation of Eccles' studies on the motoneurone.[81]

Bishop underscored both the unitary character of the nominee's work in the previous seven years and his single outstanding contributions to 'the cellular

77   Ibid, 9.
78   Ibid, 12.
79   Nomination Edinburgh 1959. Gr.II.34.
80   Ibid. Gr.II.36.
81   Nomination Whitteridge 1959.

biophysics of synaptic transmission', from the technical to the theoretical levels.[82] Eccles' collaboration with Sherrington was dropped in the second paragraph, but the really important story began with the introduction of intracellular recording in the USA and the appropriation of the technique by Eccles, who was credited with the first successful 'impalement' of a CNS neurone. 'This work', Bishop mused, 'initiated an entirely new approach to the study of synaptic transmission in the central nervous system', by making the in-vivo experiments on mammalian CNS neurones just as reliable and precise as that of 'isolated preparations of nerve and muscle'.[83] In this venture, the Australian physiologist had been supported by valuable assistants, but the nominator was sure that 'Eccles was the innovator', the one who contributed 'imagination of an extremely high order [...] experimental ingenuity, enthusiasm and sustained energy far beyond the ordinary', especially in relation to the high competition in the field by research teams of incomparable magnitude and affluence. The 'conversion' experiments were cited as the detonator of an impressive series of technical advances, experimental findings and theoretical refinements, most of which had sprung from the same laboratory in Canberra. Taken in themselves, those experiments provided the 'first direct demonstration' of the mechanism of neuronal excitation (through a depolarisation of the membrane) and 'decisive evidence' in favour of the chemical theory. The programme springing from that one 'crucial' experiment was lauded for its comprehensiveness, but especially for the introduction of ingenuous technical solutions. In this connection, the double-barrelled micropipette was given pride of place, as the key for penetrating and measuring the complex train of events leading to membrane depolarisation. Although not the place of origin of the model, Canberra was to Bishop the spring of '[n]early all our present knowledge of ionic movement at inhibitory and excitatory synapses in the spinal cord', including the physiology and anatomy of the motoneurone, the different reactivity of its component parts and their relations.[84] Many claims were still awaiting rigorous physico-chemical interpretation, also due to Eccles' habit of '[pushing] to the limit the interpretation of available experimental findings'.[85] The later work on the monosynaptic pathway was also mentioned, but only in its bearing upon the chemical theory.[86] Concluding, Bishop remarked that, mostly thanks to the candidate's own effort, 'the study of the central nervous

82   Nomination Bishop 1959. Gr.II.28.
83   Ibid, Gr.II.29.
84   Nomination Bishop 1959, Gr.II.30–31.
85   Ibid, Gr.II.31.
86   Ibid, Gr.II.32.

system has clearly been placed on an entirely new plane'.[87] In a short coda, he acknowledged Eccles' indebtedness with 'the pioneer work of the Cambridge school under the leadership of A.L. Hodgkin', and suggested 'it might be appropriate' to consider him as a joint candidate. 'Eccles', he added, 'has extended many of the ideas originally developed in connection with peripheral nerve and muscle to the *vastly more complicated situation of the motoneurons in the mammalian spinal cord*' (our emphasis), and therefore was the formal candidate.

Bernhard was entrusted with the investigation, and his concluding support to the candidature was this time untainted by doubt. He found his own 1955 objections all satisfactorily settled, thanks to the effort of Eccles himself, but also of others. Some objections still survived,[88] and it was not possible to understate Eccles' own debt with other researchers (Fatt, Katz, Hodgkin, Huxley), whose 'peripheral' results he had extended to the CNS.[89] Nevertheless, the strength of his candidacy laid in having opened the CNS to the microelectrode analysis, thus showing that this most complex system was in fact amenable to as thorough and precise an experimental study as were the more peripheral (and easier to isolate) motor axon of the squid and myoneural junction.

In 1960, there were four nominations, one from Walter Rudolf Hess (Zurich) and three from Freiburg, but no new review.[90] Nevertheless, Norrby relates of a close competition that year, between McFarlane Burnet and Peter Medawar, on the one side, and Eccles and Horace W. Magoun, on the other, proposed for their achievements on excitation and inhibition and on the reticular formation of the brain-stem, respectively.[91] Burnet and Medawar prevailed by a narrow majority, and received the Prize 'for their discovery of acquired immunological tolerance'.[92]

Eccles was once again nominated in 1961, by H.N. Robson (Medicine, University of Adelaide), 'for his discoveries of the physical-chemical mechanisms of neuro-muscular function' and by Haldan Keffer Hartline (Rockefeller Institute), 'for his discoveries elucidating the mechanisms by means of which

---

87   Ibid.
88   David P.C. Lloyd, for instance, still opposed Eccles' 'falsification' of direct inhibition in the monosynaptic pathway. Bernhard underscored that these doubts should not be underestimated, in view of the authority of the critic, who was member of an important institution and a pluri-nominee. See Review Bernhard 1959, 2; Eccles 1957.
89   Review Bernhard 1959, 7.
90   We could not find the nominations, and rely here on Norrby (2016, 97).
91   Norrby 2013; Norrby 2016.
92   By mistake, the Australian Broadcasting Corporation leaked the news of an award to Eccles, causing a wave of excitement, soon inhibited by the broadcaster's retraction.

nervous influences [...] are integrated on the surface of the nerve cell [...]'.
Robson highlighted the great value of Eccles' 'development and application of
microelectrode techniques to the intracellular investigation of nerve cells',[93]
which had encouraged others to extend the technique to cardiac, striated and
smooth muscle. Hartline focussed on his elucidation of the mechanisms of
excitation and inhibition.[94] Special emphasis was placed on Eccles' use and
refinement of 'earlier, more general ideas' (of Hodgkin and Sherrington)
and on his capacity to '[change] views on details as experimental evidence
required'. In conclusion, Hartline declared 'the new facts [Eccles had] found
and the synthesis of knowledge he has made' to constitute 'a true discovery of
lasting value to neurophysiology'.[95] The investigation this year fell on Granit,
who compiled a conjoint evaluation of Hodgkin, Huxley, Eccles and Bernhard
Katz, in consideration of the 'common core' of their researches.[96] In his section on Eccles, the reviewer mentioned his proof of a chemical mediator in
central synaptic transmission, but wished not to emphasise it. Eccles' 'great
discovery' was the demonstration and measurement of the inhibition mechanism[97] in the CNS, elevated by the technical innovations he had introduced
to the same level of control and exactness of the more 'peripheral' biophysical experiments.[98] Finally, Granit underscored how too narrow a focus on the
technical achievements or on the extension of the membrane model, did not
do justice to Eccles' grandiose theoretical edifice: thanks to his reflexological
wisdom, he had been able to get the most from a technique that, in the hand of
other researchers, had not proven a comparable source of novelty.[99] The work
of the Canberra group had not only defined an experimental standard, it had
also provided a most productive framework, thus greatly influencing succes-
sive research. In the conclusion, Granit touched upon the possible combinations for the prize, underscoring the need to give Hodgkin and Huxley priority
for the more fundamental character of their work, and showing a preference
for Eccles over Katz. The latter was 'significantly younger' and his work was
definitely 'a matter for itself'. His proposed order was then Hodgkin, Huxley
and Eccles, a subdivision remindful of the Sherrington-Adrian binomial in
1932.[100] In the session of 28 September, 1961, the Nobel Committee proposed,

---

93   Nomination Robson 1961, Gr.II.30.
94   Nomination Hartline 1961, Gr.II.31–32.
95   Ibid, Gr.II.33.
96   Review Granit 1961, 2.
97   Ibid, 12; Granit may have had some bias in this connection.
98   Ibid, 15–17.
99   Ibid, 18.
100 Ibid, 29–30.

by a 7–5 majority vote, Eccles, Hodgkin and Huxley (in this order), in recognition of 'their discovery of the ionic mechanisms of excitation and inhibition of
the membranes of peripheral and central nerve cells'.[101] A minority supported
the Hungarian Georg von Békésy, for his work on the physiology of hearing. The
Nobel Assembly followed the latter proposal.[102]

In view of the 1962 prize, Dale, Eccles' friendly foe, took the matter in his
hands.[103] In December 1961 he wrote Eccles a letter requesting help,[104] in the
form of 'a brief statement of [his] works during these relatively recent years,
which would seem to [him] to have a proper importance', and reprints. Dale's
claim was subdivided in five sections, covering Eccles' production since 1951
'and still in progress': (1) microelectrode investigations on motor nerve cells,
which elucidated the excitation mechanism; (2) Post-synaptic inhibition in its
interplay with excitation; (3) Pre-synaptic inhibition (discovered elsewhere,
'but almost the whole of its subsequent development has been due to the
researches of Eccles and his team'); (4) Chemical synaptic transmission and
pharmacology, being the confirmation of 'Dale's principle'; (5) Plasticity in the
nervous system.[105]

Dale emphasized the 'imposing continuity' and internal consistency of Eccles' production, which taken together constituted an organised attack to the
complexity of synaptic action in the CNS. He also digressed on Eccles' 'conversion', recalling how 'conspicuous' he was 'among those [...] conservatively
resistant and sceptical', how useful his criticism was to the improvement of the
chemical theory, and how Dale himself later became an enthusiastic admirer
of his unswerving scientific honesty, together with the exquisite skill and ingenuity, which Eccles devoted to new experiments of his own for testing the
possibility, which he had found so difficult to accept.[106]

But Eccles' achievement did not coincide with his simple conversion. His
extension of the chemical hypothesis, the 'convincing simplification of the approach to the solution of what may well be still regarded as one of the ultimate
problems of physiology and medicine', had 'shown a new way of access, blasted

---

101   Ibid.

102   Norrby 2013; Norrby 2016.

103   Norrby (2016) reports of several nominations for Eccles that year, which we could not
       access.

104   Dale to Eccles, 15/12/61. RSA/93/HD35.25.24. 'I need your help', he opened. 'I should like
       to have the privilege of bringing your name, and your work, to the notice of the Nobel
       committee'.

105   Dale to Members of the Nobel Prize Committee for Physiology and Medicine, 17/01/62,
       RSA/93/HD 35.25.30.

106   Ibid, 6.

a new trail' and inspired many others to follow.[107] Thus, beyond the single 'discoveries', he had shown the personality and charisma of a true man of science.

There was no investigation on Eccles for this year. Norrby, however, points at two contextual factors, which may have played against the Australian: the changing priorities following the disciplinary explosion at the Karolinska Institute in the late 1950s-early 1960s,[108] and the fact that no less than 32 physiologists were proposed that year. So, following Aarne Tiselius' suggestion, the prize took again the direction of molecular studies.[109] The 1962 Nobel Prize in Physiology or Medicine went in fact to Watson, Crick and Wilkins for their discovery of the structure of DNA. A 'due, or even overdue' prize, Dale acknowledged to Ulf von Euler after the announcement.[110] He was nevertheless unshaken in his determination to have Eccles recognised, and inquired about the procedure to renew the nomination. Which he did the following month,[111] updating the references and sharpening the motivation: [for] his work on the physiology of the nervous system, and, especially, on the modes of transmission of the nerve impulses at the synaptic junctions of the central nervous system. 'In any case', he added,

> I do not think that I need emphasize the significance of this more recent evidence for the still active progress of these immensely important investigations [...] in which Sir John Eccles has been so illustrious a pioneer.[112]

That year, Eccles was also nominated by Donald F. Magee, Professor of Pharmacology at the University of Seattle (WA), for the development of 'beautiful techniques for simultaneous stimulation of, injection of drugs into, and electrical recording from single cells within the central nervous system': the double-barrelled microelectrode. In the preamble to his report (this time limited to Hodgkin, Huxley and Eccles), Granit stressed that there was 'hardly any need for a special investigation',[113] the only matter of discussion being the prize distribution.[114] In summarising once again the achievements of the Canberra school (clear interpretation of the mechanisms of excitation and inhibition in the CNS; introduction of the double-barrelled micropipette), he only added

---

107 Ibid.
108 Norrby 2013, 236 ff.
109 Norrby 2016, 99–100.
110 Letter Dale to U.S. von Euler, 07/11/62, RSA/93/HD 35.25.24.
111 Nomination Dale 1963.
112 Ibid.
113 Review Granit 1963, 1.
114 Ibid, 10.

some more detail on pre-synaptic inhibition. As to the order of award, he fore-shadowed the possibility that Hodgkin and Huxley share the 1963 prize and Eccles be deferred to a later one (as the primacy of the Cambridge biophysi-cists both in chronological and theoretical terms was to him indisputable) but, given the beautiful convergence of the researches (excitation and inhi-bition being the phenomenon; the methods electrophysiological; the theory biophysical), and considering that the growing 'competition between different subject-groups' may deprive Eccles of a well-deserved honour, a tripartition was to be considered a 'happy solution'.[115]

In order to help the committee frame the candidates within the progress of physiological science, Granit integrated the report with the fourth chapter of his biography of Sherrington,[116] devoted to the great intuitions of the Master confirmed by later research. He admitted the frame fitted Eccles' picture better than the others', but it afforded a comprehensive view of the general problem. Saint Sherrington made the miracle. In 1963, Eccles, Hodgkin and Huxley (in this order) were finally canonised in Stockholm.

The Nature of 'Discovery'

Eccles' route to the Nobel Prize elicits a few considerations about the criteria of 'discovery', and 'benefit to mankind'. As for the latter, only one nomination (Jung 1953) established a connection between Eccles' basic science and its medical complement (the neurologist Hoffmann). All the others testify to a reductive interpretation of 'mankind' as meaning 'physiologists', and 'benefit' as 'ground-breaking advance'. Such a narrowing of the Founder's original in-tention is perhaps expected in the 1960s, after so much genetics and molecular biology. Then, we are left with the issue of 'discovery': what was Eccles nomi-nated and awarded for, and how was his 'individual' contribution framed with-in the development of physiology? On what, precisely, could Eccles be called an 'authority' of Nobel calibre? The question must be answered at two levels, of the nominators and of the reviewers, reflecting different roles and rationali-ties. Considering the nominators, no prevalent 'disciplinary' motivation for the proposals emerges from the documents we could access. In 1955, the physiolo-gist Gellhorn singled out the development of the microelectrode technique, as did the physician Robson in 1961 and the pharmacologist Magee in 1963, but all the others gave pride of place Eccles' model of excitation and inhibition. In

---

115   Ibid.
116   Granit 1966.

fact, all the nominators we have considered but one (Robson), while eventually referring to the candidate's early work, and duly dropping Sherrington's name, highlight his post-1952 achievements. In which context, the treatment of Eccles' 'conversion' to, or 'demonstration' of, chemical transmission is revealing: whereas the lengthier statements refer to it (all nominators in 1959 turn it into an ennoblement of previously 'less rigorous' ideas), only Dale singles it out, as one rubric (not the main) of his claim. The issue of authority also emerges, in particular in Bishop's 1959 statement: while acknowledging the contribution of many collaborators, as well as the incorporation of others' own 'discoveries' and ideas, he took pains to underscore how the 'innovator' was Eccles only. The recurrence of Hodgkin as co-nominee also points at the difficulty of explaining Eccles' achievements in themselves, especially as the two research programmes progressively converged in the 1950s. In this connection, contrasts between different standards of judgement interestingly emerge in 1959, with Whitteridge underscoring the 'more basic nature' and consequent greater rigour of Hodgkin's achievements, while Bishop praised Eccles' success in translating the biophysicist's original ideas in a more complex experimental system. A small number of statements (especially Dale's) also refer to Eccles' qualities as an experimentalist and scientist: his dexterity, the width and breadth of his physiological knowledge, his honesty and openness to criticism.

As to the definition of 'discovery', the few nominators who tried to single out one contribution mentioned the introduction of microelectrodes in the CNS (in which, however, Eccles' priority was disputable), the measurement of membrane potentials, or the clarification of the topology of impulse spread, which taken by themselves were not considered prize-worthy by the reviewers. Bishop (1959), Hartline (1961) and Dale (1962–63) explicitly framed the new data provided by Eccles within the 'synthesis' he had made, equating it to a discovery. By 'synthesis' they meant the model, the theory and the techniques, which had 'initiated an entirely new approach'. Finally, a few considerations meet the eye, pertaining to the character, charisma and credibility of the candidate.[117] Dale was the most explicit, but others before also praised his readiness to adjust his thought to the evidence, as well as an uncommon determination, which allowed him to beat, in so a crowded race, research centres much more central and better staffed than his own.

The reviews add two further layers of complexity: what counts as a given in evaluating scientific performance and the hierarchy of merit in the distribution of the prize. As to the first problem, the debate-at-a-distance between Granit and Bernhard on the confirmation of Eccles' model is instructive. In

---

117   See in this connection Bucchi (this volume), on the issue of 'communitarian reputation'.

1958, Granit took objection to the 1955 dismissal of the candidate's claims on grounds of insufficient consensus. Clarity was to Granit the criterion, as it would have been singular to 'deny the value of great discoveries, which means real progress', just because work was still going on in the area, and mostly under the impulse of the candidate's group. Here (discounting the deep bond of friendship between Granit and Eccles) the tension between truth and usefulness becomes palpable again: to Bernhard's attention to the single claims, Granit opposes a focus on the fate of the model in its entirety, on the stimulus and example it has provided to other researchers and groups and also (as Bishop and Dale also did) on the fact that most of the novelties introduced in this fast-developing picture came from Eccles' own lab, despite worldwide competition. In the last review, Granit stressed the wholeness of Eccles' achievement, independent from single experimental claims.

As to the second point, it emerged in the last two collective reviews, in which prize-worthiness was no more an issue, but primacy was. On both occasions (1961 and 1963) the reviewer was Granit, and he reiterated the persuasion that Hodgkin and Huxley deserved either chronological or order- priority, in view of the more basic and exact nature of their achievements, and the greatest experimental rigour their system allowed. This seems more an epistemological yardstick, than anything related to 'benefit to mankind': in the comparison between an isolated system from a phylogenetically distant model and a whole-animal vertebrate system more complicated and less elegant, but arguably closer to its possible medical target, the first is preferred for the greater control of the variables it affords.[118] Such an assessment appears also to contrast with a different angle, occasionally expressed by the nominators and both the reviewers: namely, the greater difficulty of Eccles' problem, and the greater skill, ingenuity and physiological wisdom required to solve it.

Enacting Authority. Eccles as a Nobelist

A good ten years older than his co-recipients, Eccles had still a decade of active research after canonisation. This allows us to attempt an analysis of three more facets of authority. First is the idea, well put by Duffin in this volume, that 'laureates find themselves expatiating on topics for which they have no expertise, including philosophy and politics'. Second is the extent of Eccles' own perception of himself as belonging to a new élite, and whether this made him

---

118   One of us has observed how these remarks add one further layer of complexity to the
        centre-periphery relations in the history of science.

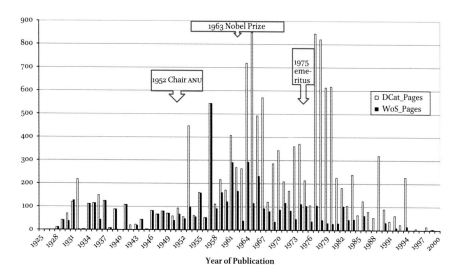

FIGURE 7.1   Total number of pages published by John C. Eccles (journals or books).
SOURCES: DÜSSELDORF LIBRARY CATALOGUE. SEE ALSO PIEPER-SCHOLZ
ET AL. 2011

more prone to take fellow-Nobel Prizes on board as authorities. Finally, we will inquire whether the perception of Eccles by his peers was in any way changed by the Nobel Prize, again through citation analysis.

We consider Eccles' publishing and citation behaviour in roughly two decades before and after the Nobel (between 1952 – 'conversion' and move to the ANU, and his retirement in 1975), as well as the eventual changes in recognition of his own work stemming from the citation behaviour of colleagues.[119] In the period covered (1952–74) Eccles published two thirds of all his works, 442 articles, books, edited books or chapters (over a total of 642 listed in Freund et al. 2011. See Figure 7.1), which confirms his fame as a mighty productive writer. As to the topics covered (Figure 7.2), the 'imposing continuity' praised by Dale is confirmed. Throughout the period, in fact, he never ceased publishing on 'his' topics (here subsumed under neurophysiology), and the rise of papers on the brain-stem after 1964 (although here separated from the classic spinal cord work) are safely regarded as an extension of his original approach, as to theoretical framework and method. The only major change we observe, apparently supporting Duffin's claim of post-Nobel 'expatiation' of Nobelists, is the increase of Eccles' writings on Mind-body relations, as well as on cultural evolution and Popper's philosophy (subsumed under 'Humanities').

---

119   A caveat is here due about the tentative nature of our scrutiny.

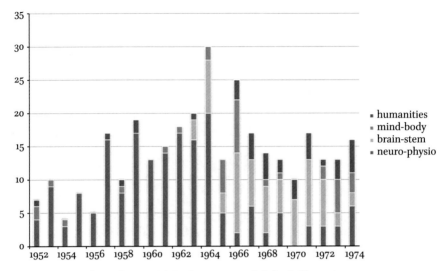

FIGURE 7.2   Yearly production, J.C. Eccles, 1952–1974. Subdivided by major areas

Nevertheless, here the quantitative approach is fruitfully corrected by qualitative considerations. If these topics only appear sporadically before 1964, it is worth highlighting that the one 1953 publication in the field was the book *The Neurophysiological Basis of the Mind. The Principles of Neurophysiology* , Eccles' first attempt at providing a system of cellular neurophysiology.[120] In that book, Descartes, Sherrington and Popper alternate with membrane constants, anatomical considerations and micrographs to make the case for a dualist physiology as 'Science of Man'. It was the lack of recognition for the truly scientific character of this attempt that started what Eccles called his 'Long Interregnum', during which, however, he kept thinking and publicly speaking about the mind/body issue.[121] Our very separation of the Mind/body and Humanities categories may be regarded as artificial, as one of the consequences of Eccles' philosophical conversion was exactly the attempt at giving Cartesian dualism the shape of a proper scientific hypothesis, as attested by the study-week he organised in 1964 for the Pontificia Academia Scientiarum.[122] The problem, here, is that his concept of the relations between religion, culture, politics and

---

120   Eccles 1953. The book was preceded in 1951 by an article on Nature (Eccles 1951) on his own Popperian hypothesis of mind/brain relations, which fell outside the scope of our review. On the book, Shepherd comments (arguably without irony): 'For a young medical student in the 1950s determined to become a neurophysiologist, it was, if not the tablets of Moses, something close to them'. (Shepherd 2009, 94).

121   Eccles 1994, 17.

122   Eccles 1966a.

science diverged from the neat separation we consider typical of the scientist.[123] Here again, the punctual impressions have to be studiously contextualised: it is possible that Eccles' philosophy was a bad one, but it was an earnest attempt at doing science as he thought it was. On the other hand, some fellow-travellers in these philosophical/scientific adventures made much out of his Laureate status (e.g. Sun Myung Moon's Unification Church or the parapsychologists[124]), just as they did before with his titles of Sir or Fellow of the Royal Society.

As to the citation behaviour, we tested whether Eccles' post-Nobel publications contain an enhanced number of references to laureates than his earlier papers, as a possible sign of his renovated self-perception as member of an élite. Here, in addition to 80 scientific articles from the decade before, and 83 from after the prize (i.e. those present in the Web Of Science database), we directly compared a 1961 review[125] on synaptic transmission with the book *The physiology of Synapses*, which was an expansion of it, presented on the occasion of the award ceremony,[126] and which contained almost twice as many references and referenced authors (roughly one-fourth of the added references only was due to updates. See Table 7.1). Both comparisons have born essentially negative results (Table 7.2).[127] There is even a decrease in citations of Nobelists, both in comprehensive reviews (columns 3–4) and in research papers (column 2 vs 5), and pioneer papers were given more credit than their recent articles. Actually, Eccles' post-prize production even shows a considerable decrease in individual citations of Nobelists, with slight exceptions of Adrian and Eccles himself. This self-citation behaviour, also varying between original and review articles, remains almost stable due to be the centrality of Eccles' group within their domain of research, as well as the complexity of the research programme, which forced the researchers to work on each and every level of the problem (anatomy, physiology, chemistry etc.) in order to provide a clear picture. It is the steady development of Eccles' experimental system, his own question-producing machine, what can most likely explain this behaviour.

---

123 See Eccles 1947; Eccles 1970; Eccles 1979; Eccles 1980.

124 See also Cousins 1985.

125 Eccles 1961.

126 Eccles 1964.

127 By the way, the mentioned review article in *Ergebnisse der Physiologie* 1961 which cited 426 titles was cited only 159 times by other articles in the database, after a little increase there was soon stagnation and a sharp decrease since 1965. Whereas the increase eventually points at some 'Nobel effect', this review article soon came into competition with the 1964 monograph, which like almost every book not included in the Web of Science database.

TABLE 7.1   Comparison (Eccles 1961) as Non-Nobelist vs (Eccles 1964) as Nobelist review
author

Publication	Review Ergebnisse 1961	Monograph Springer 1964
References (Refs.) TOTAL	426 (43% of monograph)	997
First authors of refs.	178 (48% of monograph)	374
Refs. 1961	10	104
Refs. 1962	—	105
Refs. 1963	—	60
Refs. in print	0	10
Additional refs. as update 1961–64	—	269 (27%)
Additional refs. to enhance content	—	302 (30%)

Summing up, the Nobel Prize does not seem to us to have added anything substantial to Eccles' self-representation as an élite scientist. He had this conviction before and, consistent with his sense of the importance of tradition in science,[128] he derived it from his own academic ancestry and from the intrinsic nobleness of the branch of science he cultivated. We do not mean to belittle the subjective importance of the award to him, but just to point out that he possibly saw it as a consequence, and enhancement, of an authority rooted in the long history of physiology since Descartes.[129] A hint in this direction is provided by the introduction to his 1964 book, in which he acknowledged 'the influence of three great scientists as [he had] striven to give a coherent account of the synapses: Ramon y Cajal (anatomy), Sherrington (physiology) and Dale (pharmacology)'.[130] It was a due homage to three great men (and Nobel laureates), as well as an implicit statement that amid such wisdom he was fourth. As to Sherrington, the continuity that Eccles perceived between himself and the Master stems clearly from his Nobel speech. On December 11th, 1963 (31 years after Sherrington had lectured on 'Inhibition as a coordinative factor', Sherrington 1932) Eccles spoke on 'The ionic mechanism of postsynaptic inhibition'.[131] All the critical elements of a decade-long adventure were summarised: the revised chemistry, biophysics, anatomy and topology

---

128   Eccles 1947; Eccles 1970, 134.
129   Eccles 1953.
130   Interestingly, no mention is made of Popper.
131   Eccles 1964.

TABLE 7.2   Citations of Nobel Laureates by Eccles in: 1. scientific articles 1952–52 (column 2); Eccles 1961 (col. 3); Eccles 1964 (col. 4); scientific articles 1964–74 (column 5); in contrast citations of Eccles by Laureates 1952–62 vs 1964–74 (col. 6). Columns 2, 5 and 6 from Thomson Reuters' ISI Web of Science Core Collection

Nobelist (chronol.)	80 articles 1952–62	Review 1961	Monograph 1964	83 articles 1964–74	Eccles cited before vs after 1963
Golgi (NP 1906, d. 1926)	0	0	3[a]	0	0
Adrian (NP 1932, d. 1977)	3	3	3[a]	4	0
Sherrington (NP 1932, d. 1952)	4	1	6[a]	0	0
Dale (NP 1936, d. 1968)	2	0	7[a]	1	0
Loewi (NP 1936, d. 1961)	0	0	5[a]	0	0
Gasser (NP 1944, d. 1963)	0	1	3[a]	0	0
Robbins (NP 1954, d. 2003)	0	1	2[a]	0	0
Bovet (NP 1961, d. 1992)	1	0	0	1[a]	2 : 0
Eccles (NP 1963)	*120*	*48*	95 [b]38 post 1960	111	120 : 111
Hodgkin (NP 1963)	*17*	*6*	5[a]	4[a]	1 : 0
Huxley (NP 1963)	*11*	*1*	1[a]	1[a]	1 : 1[a]
Granit (NP 1967)	*16*	*4*	*11* [b]2	3[a]	12 : 14 [b]4
Axelrod (NP 1970)	*0*	*0*	*1*[a]	0	0
Euler U.v. (NP 1970)	*1*	*1*	3[a]	0	0
Katz (NP 1970)	*19*	*27*	35 [b]3	8 [b]1	8 : 3 [b]1
Hubel (NP 1981)	*1*	*0*	*0*	4	0
Sperry (NP 1981)	5	*1*	9[a]	6	*1* : 2 [b]2
Wiesel (NP 1981)	0	2	*0*	4	0
Articles cited	608	426	997	580	
Self-citations	19.7%	11.3%	9.5%	19.1%	
Other Nobelists cited	13.2%	11.3%	9.4%	6.2%	

a   no citation of articles published after 1960.
b   portion of articles published after 1960.

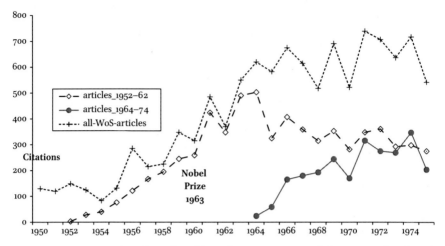

FIGURE 7.3   Citations of articles authored by Eccles as senior Non-Nobelist 1952–62 (h-index 53) vs articles by the Nobel lab researcher 1964–74 (h-index 38) vs all citations 1929–75.
DATA SOURCE: WEB OF SCIENCE CORE COLLECTION [8.6.2017]

of the nerve cell, the technical breakthroughs, the 'fortunate choice' of moto-neurones, Hodgkin's membrane model and ion pump. Not a single mention of Sherrington throughout the paper. And yet, it is difficult not to speculate about the intimate relation between the two speeches, so much different in tone and breadth. Whereas Sherrington had kept his argument much shorter, easier to understand, had duly contextualised his own achievements in the history of the subject, and had closed on the possible medical significance of inhibition, Eccles' lecture read like a scientific paper: dry, highly technical, with little con-cessions to rhetoric. Still, from the title ('The mechanism...'), to the conclusion ('thus effecting inhibition'), all the Lecture reads as a vindication of the theory Sherrington could only present in tentative terms (inhibition 'seems' to be ubiq-uitous; co-ordination 'appears' to be outcome of a nice adjustment; the mecha-nisms of excitation and inhibition put in quotation marks). There is no need for much contextualisation or reference to medicine when you have science at its best – neurophysiology, the 'Science of Man',[132] the physics of the biological sciences, now re-founded on the pillar of its central mechanism: inhibition.

   As to Eccles' perception by his peers, what can be gathered from citation analysis seems to rule out any notable Nobel-effect (Tab. 7.2 column 6; compare Chan 2014).[133] At least some slight enhancement and consolidation can be traced in the Web of Science: Figure 7.3 compares the citation scores (to 1997) of

132   Eccles 1953.
133   Although an attempt to predict Nobel Prize Winners by means of Garfield's citation database listed Eccles on rank 22 of the most cited scientists until 1967 with just 4

81 articles published by Eccles between 1952 and 1962 to 83 in the post-Nobel decade as portions of the total. Articles published in the period 1964–74 as Nobelist became only in 1974 more cited than those published in the previous decade and contributed less to his impact than pre-Nobel publications.[134]

Conclusion

This case-study can be considered exemplary of post-WWII trends, like the enhanced perception of basic science and of its medical import, the increased difficulty in singling out a 'discovery' or a 'discoverer' following the quantitative explosion of organised research, and the constantly shifting criteria of evaluation. Nevertheless, we are left with the legitimate suspicion that similar mechanisms may have been at work before in the history of the Nobel Prize in Physiology or Medicine (Sherrington would be a case to investigate more closely, as well as Golgi and Cajal), and that very little confidence can be cast on any epoch-making watershed one would care to introduce. A different, larger-scale approach would be more effective in this connection.

As to the three instances of authority (in the making; during the evaluation; after being awarded) we have argued (following Borck[135]) that the greatest determinant of Eccles' rise in authority within his communities of reference was the potential of his experimental system, and the questions it engendered were more relevant than the answers it afforded. As far as the assessment of authority is concerned, the co-evolution of the criteria with the maturation of the experimental system has emerged, as well as the complex interplay of the primary criterion (discovery benefiting mankind) with contingent standards, wherein the former is reinterpreted but not obliterated. We have shown how, even in this case, the temptation of awarding 'achievements' in general, instead than 'discovery' in particular, has been resisted. Contrary to what the otherwise excellent Casey has argued (on the basis of Dale's 1962 nomination, only, and of a suggestion by Eccles' old associate William Gibson), the Nobel

---

Nobelists scoring higher than him (Garfield 1970, fig. 3), this effect cannot be repeated in the actual database which has grown tremendously since then, the Web of Science Core Collection lists 24.259 citations altogether and calculates Eccles' Hirsch-index as 86. Thus, our historical analysis was limited to the time-span of Eccles scientific life 1927–97.

134 Cf. also Citation Report for Eccles JC* via http://apps.webofknowledge.com (February 26, 2019).

135 Borck 2017.

prize to Eccles was not a 'career' prize.[136] The point is rather that in this case we need to critically reassess our naïve concept of 'discovery'.

Acknowledgements

The authors are grateful to Chantal Marazia for her invaluable assistance with (and criticism of) this chapter at various stages; to Cornelius Borck for his generosity with both encouragement and criticism. Files on Eccles in the Nobel Prize archive were kindly provided by the Nobel Committee for Physiology or Medicine.

Bibliography

Bacq, Z.M. 1974. *Chemical transmission of nerve impulses: a historical sketch*. Oxford: Pergamon Press.

Barthes, R. 1981. *Camera Lucida: Reflections on Photography*. Translated by Richard Howard. New York: Hill and Wang.

Bennett, M.R. 2001. *History of the Synapse*. Amsterdam: Harwood Academic.

Bennett, M. 1985. 'Nicked by Occam's razor: unitarianism in the investigation of synaptic transmission'. *The Biological Bulletin*, 168 (3S): 159–167.

Borck, C. 1998. 'John C. Eccles (1903–1997): Neurophysiologist and Neurophilosopher'. *Journal of the History of the Neurosciences* (71): 76–81.

Borck, C. 2017. 'Soups and Sparks Revisited'. *Nuncius* 32 (2): 286–329.

Brock, L.G.; Coombs, J.S.; Eccles, J.C. 1952. 'The recording of potentials from motoneurones with an intracellular electrode'. *The Journal of Physiology* 117(4): 431–460.

Brock, L.G.; Coombs, J.S.; Eccles, J.C. 1952. 'Antidromic propagation of impulses into motoneurones'. In *The Spinal Cord. Ciba Foundation Symposium*, edited by John Laurence Malcolm, 120–131. London: Churchill.

Brooks, C. 1958. 'Current developments in thought and the past evolution of ideas concerning integrative function'. In *The History and Philosophy of Knowledge of the Brain and its Functions*, edited by Frederick Noel Lawrence Poynter, 235–252. Oxford: Blackwell.

Brooks, C. and Eccles, J.C. 1947. 'An electrical hypothesis of central inhibition'. *Nature* 159 (4049): 760–764.

Cannon, W.B. 1939. 'The argument for chemical mediation of nerve impulses'. *Science* 90 (2345): 521–527.

---

136   Casey 2009.

Casey, B.P. 2009. 'Against the materialists: John Carew Eccles, Karl Raimund Popper and the ghost in the machine'. Yale: Yale University.

Coombs, J.S.; Curtis, D.R.; Eccles, J.C. 1959. 'The electrical constants of the motoneurone membrane'. *The Journal of physiology* 145 (3): 505–528.

Coombs, J.S.; Eccles, J.C.; Fatt, P. 1953. 'The action of the inhibitory synaptic transmitter'. *Australian Journal of Science* 16: 1–5.

Coombs, J.S.; Eccles, J.C.; Fatt, P. 1955. 'The specific ionic conductances and the ionic movements across the motoneuronal membrane that produce the inhibitory postsynaptic potential'. *The Journal of physiology* 130 (2): 326–373.

Cousins, N. 1985. *Nobel Prize Conversations with Sir John Eccles, Roger Sperry, Ilya Prigogine, Brian Josephson.* San Francisco: Saybrook.

Curtis, D.R. and Andersen, P. 2001. 'Sir John Carew Eccles, A.C. 27 January 1903–2 May 1997'. *Biographical Memoirs of Fellows of the Royal Society* 47: 161–187.

Dale, H.H. 1954. 'The beginnings and prospects of neurohumoral transmission'. *Pharmacological Reviews* 6 (1): 7–13.

Dupont, J.C. 1999. *Histoire de la Neurotransmission.* Paris: Presses Universitaires de France.

Eccles, J.C. 1937. 'Synaptic and neuro-muscular transmission'. *Physiological Reviews* 17 (4): 538–555.

Eccles, J.C. 1945. 'An electrical hypothesis of synaptic and neuromuscular transmission'. *Nature* 156 (3971): 680–683.

Eccles, J.C. 1946. 'An electrical hypothesis of synaptic and neuro-muscular transmission'. *Annals of the New York Academy of Sciences* 47 (1): 429–455.

Eccles, J.C. 1947. 'Man and Freedom'. *Twentieth Century* 2: 5–23.

Eccles, J.C. 1951. 'Hypotheses Relating to the Brain–Mind Problem'. *Nature* 168 (4263): 53–57.

Eccles, J.C. 1952. 'The electrophysiological properties of the motoneurone'. *Cold Spring Harbor Symposia on Quantitative Biology* 17: 175–183.

Eccles, J.C. 1953. *The Neurophysiological Basis of Mind: The Principles of Neurophysiology. The Waynflete Lectures, 1952.* Oxford: Clarendon Press.

Eccles, J.C. 1957. *The Physiology of Nerve Cells. The Herter Lectures, 1955.* Baltimore: Johns Hopkins University Press.

Eccles, J.C. 1964a. 'Ionic Mechanism of Postsynaptic Inhibition'. *Science* 145(3637): 1140–1147.

Eccles, J.C. 1964b. *The Physiology of Synapses.* Berlin: Springer

Eccles, J.C. 1966. 'Some observations on the strategy of neurophysiological research'. In *Nerve as a tissue,* edited by Kaare Rodahl and Bela Issekutz Jr., 445–456. New York: Harper & Row.

Eccles, J.C. (ed.) 1966a. *Brain and conscious experience. Study week Sept. 28 to Oct. 4, 1964, of the Pontificia Academia Scientiarum.* New York: Springer.

Eccles, J.C. 1970. *Facing Reality: Philosophical adventures by a brain scientist*. Basel: Roche (in collaboration with Springer Verlag).

Eccles, J.C. 1974. 'The world of objective knowledge'. In *The philosophy of Karl Popper*, edited by Paul Arthur Schilpp, 349–370. Open Court: La Salle.

Eccles, J.C. 1975. 'Under the spell of the synapse'. In *The Neurosciences: Paths of Discovery*, edited by Frederick G. Worden, Judith P. Swazey; George Adelman, 159–180. Cambridge (Mass.): MIT Press.

Eccles, J.C. 1976. 'From Electrical to Chemical Transmission in the Central Nervous System'. *Notes and Records of the Royal Society of London* 30 (2): 219–230.

Eccles, J.C. 1977. 'My scientific odyssey'. *Annual review of physiology* 39 (1): 1–20.

Eccles, J.C. 1979. *The Human Mystery (Gifford Lectures 1977–1978)*. Berlin: Springer.

Eccles, J.C. 1980. *The Human Psyche (Gifford Lectures 1978–1979)*. Berlin: Springer.

Eccles, J.C. 1982. 'The synapse: from electrical to chemical transmission'. *Annual Review of Neuroscience* 5 (1): 325–339.

Eccles, J.C. 1982a. 'Life in Sherrington's laboratory: his last decade at Oxford 1925–1935'. *Trends in Neurosciences* 5: 108–110.

Eccles, J.C. 1987. 'The story of the Renshaw cell'. In *Neurobiology of acetylcholine. Proceedings of a symposium held in honor of Alexander G. Karczmar, June 5–7, 1985, in Maywood Ill*, edited by Nae J. Dun and Robert L. Perlman, 189–194. New York/London: Plenum.

Eccles, J.C. 1994. *How the Self controls its Brain*. Berlin: Springer.

Feldberg, W. 1977. 'Acetylcholine: Reminiscences of an Eye Witness'. In *The Pursuit of Nature: Informal Essays on the History of Physiology*, edited by Alan Lloyd Hodgkin, 65–83. Cambridge: Cambridge University Press.

Fillenz, M. 2000. 'Memories of Sir John Eccles in New Zealand'. In *Sir John Eccles in Memoriam—A Tireless Warrior for Dualism*, edited by Helena Eccles and Hans-Jürgen Biersack, 11–28. Landsberg: Ecomed.

Fillenz, M. 2012. 'Memories of John Eccles'. *Journal of the History of the Neurosciences* 21 (2): 214–226.

Freund, Hans-Joachim, Koppitz, U.; Labisch, A.E. (eds.) 2011. *The Legacy of John C. Eccles – Selected letters (1937–1963) and guide to the archive in Düsseldorf*. Aachen: Shaker Verlag.

Garfield, E. 1970. 'Citation indexing for studying science'. *Nature* 227 (5259): 669–671.

Girolami, P.; Taborikova, H.; Nistico, G. (eds.) 1994. *In Memory of Sir Henry Dale*. Reana del Rojale: Chiandetti.

Granit, R. 1966. *Charles Scott Sherrington: An Appraisal*. London: Nelson.

Gross, C. 2013. 'Some revolutions in neuroscience'. *Journal of cognitive neuroscience* 25 (1): 4–13.

Hebb, D.O. 1961. 'Distinctive features of learning in the higher animal'. In *Brain mechanisms and learning*, edited by Alfred Fessard, Ralph Waldo Gerard, Jerzy Konorski; Jean-Francois Delafresnaye, 37–46. Oxford: Clarendon.

Jacobson, M. 2013. *Foundations of neuroscience*. New York: Springer Science & Business Media.

Karczmar, A.G. 2001. 'Sir John Eccles, 1903–1997. Part 1. Onto the demonstration of the chemical nature of transmission in the CNS'. *Perspectives in biology and medicine* 44 (1): 76–86.

Katz, Bernard. 1996. '[Autobiographical Sketch]'. *The History of Neuroscience in Autobiography* 1: 350–381. Washington: Society for Neuroscience.

Marcum, J.A. 2006. "Soups" vs. 'Sparks': Alexander Forbes and the synaptic transmission controversy'. *Annals of science* 63 (2): 139–156.

McIntyre, A.K. 1954. 'Central and sensory transmission'. *Pharmacological Reviews* 6 (1): 103–104.

Merton, R.K. 1973. 'Recognition and excellence: instructive ambiguities'. In *RK Merton, The sociology of science. Theoretical and empirical investigations*, edited by Norman W. Storer, 419–437. Chicago: University of Chicago Press.

Norrby, E. 2013. *Nobel Prizes and Nature's Surprises*. Singapore: World Scientific.

Norrby, E. 2016. *Nobel Prizes and Notable Discoveries*. Singapore: World Scientific.

Pieper-Scholz, I.; Isberner, C.; Koppitz, U. 2011. 'Catalogue raisonné of publications by John C. Eccles'. In *The Legacy of John C. Eccles – Selected letters (1937–1963) and guide to the archive in Düsseldorf*, edited by Hans-Joachim Freund, Ulrich Koppitz; Alfons Eberhard Labisch, 33–83. Aachen: Shaker Verlag.

Rheinberger, H.J. 1997. *Toward a History of Epistemic Things: Synthesizing Proteins in the Test Tube*. Stanford (CA): Stanford University Press.

Robinson, J.D. 2001. *Mechanisms of synaptic transmission: bridging the gaps (1890–1990)*. Oxford: Oxford University Press.

Shaw, F.H. 1954. 'Transmission and block in sympathetic ganglia'. *Pharmacological Reviews* 6 (1): 69–70.

Shepherd, G.M. 2008. 'Eccles, John Carew'. In *New Dictionary of Scientific Biography*, edited by Noretta Koertge, 329–333. New York: Charles Scribner's Sons.

Shepherd, G.M. 2009. *Creating modern neuroscience: the revolutionary 1950s*. Oxford: Oxford University Press.

Sherrington, C.S. 1932. 'Inhibition as a coordinative factor'. In *Nobel Lectures, Physiology and Medicine*: 278–289.

Sherrington, C.S. 1906. *The Integrative Action of the Nervous System*. New York: Charles Scribner's Sons.

Smith, R. 1992. *Inhibition: History and meaning in the sciences of mind and brain*. Los Angeles: University of California Press.

Smith, R. 2000. 'The embodiment of value: CS Sherrington and the cultivation of science'. *The British Journal for the History of Science* 33 (3): 283–311.

Smith, R. 2001. 'Representations of mind: CS Sherrington and scientific opinion, c. 1930–1950'. *Science in Context* 14 (4): 511–539.

Smith, R. 2003. 'Biology and values in interwar Britain: CS Sherrington, Julian Huxley and the vision of progress'. *Past & Present* 178: 210–242.

Stuart, D.G. and Brownstone, R.M. 2011. 'The beginning of intracellular recording in spinal neurons: facts, reflections, and speculations'. *Brain research* 1409: 62–92.

Stuart, D.G. and Pierce, P.A. 2006. 'The academic lineage of Sir John Carew Eccles (1903–1997)'. *Progress in Neurobiology* 78 (3–5): 136–155.

Todes, D.P. 2002. *Pavlov's physiology factory: Experiment, interpretation, laboratory enterprise*. Baltimore: Johns Hopkins University Press.

Todman, D. 2008. 'John Eccles (1903–97) and the experiment that proved chemical synaptic transmission in the central nervous system'. *Journal of Clinical Neuroscience* 15(9): 972–977.

Valenstein, E.S. 2002. 'The discovery of chemical neurotransmitters'. *Brain and cognition* 49(1): 73–95.

Valenstein, E.S. 2006. *The war of the soups and the sparks: The discovery of neurotransmitters and the dispute over how nerves communicate*. New York: Columbia University Press.

CHAPTER 8

The Laureate in the Spotlight: Renato Dulbecco and the Public Image of Science

Massimiano Bucchi

This chapter focuses on the 1999 participation of Medicine laureate Renato Dulbecco (1975) in one of the most popular Italian TV shows: the broadcast of the Sanremo Festival music competition. Through an analysis of the show, its media coverage and an empirical study of public opinion conducted in its aftermath, the chapter focuses on the implications of the laureate's TV appearance for the public image of the Nobel Prize laureates and of scientists. More broadly, it also describes how this TV appearance resonates with some of the dominant popular narratives characterizing public discourse on the Nobel.

The Nobel Prize and the Public Image of Science

'Dad, all my friends think this is so cool!'. Thus Peter Agre's children welcomed their father after the news spread that he had received the Nobel Prize for chemistry 2003. 'In my whole life since my kids became teenagers, this is the first time they've come home and said [that]', remarked the scientist, understanding that he had passed the threshold beyond which scientific reputation transforms itself into media visibility and even celebrity.[1]

This and related dynamics were described by the founder of the sociology of science, Robert K. Merton, as the 'Matthew effect', from the passage in Matthew's Gospel which states, 'For unto every one that hath shall be given, and he shall have abundance: but from him that hath not shall be taken away even that which he hath'.[2] Those in positions of visibility and prestige will have privileged access to further resources and positions. As a Nobel Prize winner for physics once put it, 'The world is peculiar in this matter of how it gives credit. It tends to give the credit to [already] famous people'.[3]

---

1   Cited in Pratt 2012, 41.
2   Matthew 25:29.
3   Merton 1973, 443.

Although Merton originally referred mainly to dynamics within the scientific community, several studies have shown later that this effect not only extends to scientists' visibility in society at large but also amplifies and connects with general media and public discourse dynamics. Thus, the high reputation of certain scientists (as certified by the Nobel Prize and other particularly prestigious forms of recognition) is transformed into a visibility which exceeds the esteem of peers, turning them into all-round celebrities, not dissimilar to sports or media personalities.[4]

Studying the visibility of Nobel laureates in the sciences is an extraordinary gateway for understanding transformations in the public image of science – and of scientists – throughout the 20th century and also understanding how the Prize itself contributed to shape such image. The Nobel Prize announcements are in fact one of the occasions when science makes global headlines in the media. The halo and reputation of the Prize are reaching even those audiences which are quite distant and not much interested in science. In fiction – from Hollywood movies to the Simpsons – 'Nobel' has become a metonym for brilliant minds, genius and successful science. According to data of the Science in Society Monitor, a yearly survey of Italian citizens' perception of and attitudes towards science, 85% of Italians know what the Nobel Prize is. As Harriet Zuckerman (1996 [1977]) noted in her book *Scientific Elite*:

> I am inclined to think that the principal effect of the Prize on science in the large is indirect; its influence on the public's image of science probably counts for more than its function as incentive for scientific accomplishment. Decades-long reiterated attention to the Prizes and the laureates in the public press, to their great achievements and to the ceremony honoring them, announces to the public that great things are stirring in science, things worthy of public admiration and public support.[5]

In this scenario, Nobel laureates can become valuable communicative resources that can be employed, not only on science matters. To the media they represent the possibility of personalizing themes and complex issues, as well as anchoring and ennobling the most diverse topics to the prestige of the Prize and its protagonists. News media ask Nobel laureates for their opinion and advice on a striking variety of matters. 'Levi Montalcini: less cars, more buses', titled the newspaper *Corriere della Sera* on 9 November 1986, referring to an

---

4 Bucchi 2015; Fahy 2015; Fahy and Lewenstein 2014; Goodell 1977; Zuckerman 1996 [1977].
5 Zuckerman 1996 [1977], xxviii.

interview on Rome's traffic problems with the scientist, who had just received the Nobel prize for Medicine.

This use of the Nobel laureate as a cornerstone of authority, rhetorical resource and source of prestige to legitimate certain positions – and not just scientific ones – is particularly common in the media. Such use characterizes a relevant proportion of articles citing Nobel laureates in the daily press.[6] A typical case of this 'use' of Nobel laureates in the media would be to mention their position with regard to a certain initiative, controversial theme, emerging issue loosely connected with the domains of science and technology. To give just a few examples:

> Nobel laureate Renato Dulbecco, the father of the Genome, approves the initiative of the US President and the UK Prime Minister on the Genome Project.[7]
> Yes from two Nobel laureates to euthanasia.[8]
> Xenotransplants are not new, but if Nobel laureate Renato Dulbecco, gives his support, one could nourish hope that all of this will soon become real.[9]
> More than 100 of Britain's top medical scientists, including five Nobel Prize winners, have launched an attack on red tape in research which, they say, is allowing rivals in other countries to race ahead.[10]
> [...] letter signed by 110 of the country's most eminent medical researchers, including five Nobel Prize winners and 38 Fellows of the Royal Society.[11]

The name of Nobel laureates is also employed by news media to confirm to the reader the relevance of a certain initiative or institution:

> An institution that boasted among its members the Nobel laureate for chemistry Giulio Natta.[12]
> The Prize was given by the President of the Jury James Black, Nobel Prize for medicine in 1988.[13]

---

6   Beltrame 2007.
7   Corriere della Sera, 16 march 2000.
8   Corriere della Sera 6 December 2000.
9   Corriere della Sera 8 September 2001.
10   The Times 13 June 2000.
11   The Times 13 June 2000.
12   Corriere della Sera 29 June 2001.
13   Corriere della Sera 20 February 2001.

The celebrity of Nobel laureates, not unlike those of other show business personalities familiar to the general public, reverberates also on other initiatives
and social events that bear no relation with science:

> Nobel laureate in medicine [Rita Levi Montalcini], sitting in the first row
> in her unfailing black velvet dress.[14]
> Much admired two great personalities. The Nobel laureate Rita Levi
> Montalcini (in a shiny elegant black dress) and dancer Carla Fracci (in
> delicate white trousers).[15]

This 'halo effect' of the Nobel laureate extends to a variety of situations also
beyond media coverage. Thus for instance, the presence of a Nobel laureate
on the board of a hi-tech company can become a resource of legitimation; his/
her visit to a research institution or the support of a charity campaign can have
impact on the visibility of institutions or initiatives; and even make its entry
into the history of entertainment, as it happened at the end of the 1990s with
Renato Dulbecco as presenter of the Sanremo Festival.

A Nobel at the Sanremo Song Festival

Who knows whether Alfred Nobel, having established his residence in Sanremo during the last years of his life, could ever have imagined the curious
situation that involved one of 'his' laureates about a century later. Since 1951,
Sanremo hosts the 'Festival della canzone Italiana', a competition among singers performing original songs that has historically been a key media event –
its live broadcast over several evenings reaching an audience that has peaked
with 16 million viewers and almost 70% TV audience share. The mid-90s editions, however, had not been very successful.[16]

When the 49th edition started on 23 February 1999, the main presenter Fabio Fazio and the French model Laetitia Casta were joined on stage by Nobel
laureate in medicine 1975 Renato Dulbecco.[17] Dulbecco explained his decision of accepting the invitation as follows: 'I thought that a scientist on the

---

14   Corriere della Sera, 8 October 2001.
15   Corriere della Sera, 29 march 2001.
16   On the general history of Sanremo Festival see Anselmi 2009.
17   Renato Dulbecco (1914–2012) shared the 1975 medicine Prize with David Baltimore and
      Howard Temin 'for their discoveries concerning the interaction between tumor viruses
      and the genetic material of the cell'.

Festival stage would do *propaganda for science*' (italics mine).[18] However, during the Festival and its related media exposure, Dulbecco actually spoke very little about science in general and even less about his own research. Even in interviews with the press questions touched more on his life experience in the US, on his personal relationships with other famous science personalities like Rita Levi Montalcini – another Nobel laureate in medicine, 1986 – with whom Dulbecco confessed to have fallen in love when he was younger, on his musical tastes and how he was preparing to live the Sanremo experience. During one of the interviews before the Festival, Dulbecco also mentioned a personal connection with the Festival location: it was from Sanremo that he left for his military duty in the Second World War.

No mention is even made of the contribution for which Dulbecco received the prestigious Prize established by Alfred Nobel. His Nobel contribution is vaguely mentioned as 'a discovery that helped finding a vaccine for poliomyelitis'. TV and daily news often emphasized his good physical shape despite his age (85 at the time), his brilliant conversation and wit. During the Festival, Dulbecco mostly limited himself to introducing some singers on stage, exchanging a few words with the other presenters, Fabio Fazio and Laetitia Casta, and taking part in the Prize awarding ceremony once the Festival winners were announced. Only during the final evening, he briefly mentioned the hopes that can be reasonably nurtured for the future progress of cancer research and the need to support it. On that occasion, he also mentioned his intention to donate his own earnings from the Festival to cancer research.

The presence and role of Dulbecco during the Festival unfolded between two widespread 'popular narratives' of the scientist and his role in society.[19] According to the first narrative, the scientist is 'someone special', 'different from the rest of us': a genius, somebody who sees what we ignore and who has been able to reach where we cannot. According to the second narrative, the scientist, even if s/he is a Nobel laureate, still remains 'a normal person, one of us'. In this case, the image of science and its protagonists is more reassuring and closer to the general public. It is not the image of the scientist manipulating genes and building uncontrollable apparatuses, but rather the scientist that works hard day by day with modesty, humility and patience and presents himself as a model within reach for anybody having the good will to engage in study and research. A similar tension was identified by studies of Nobel laureates in other television contexts, 'instantiating the tension the Nobel Prize encapsulates between the recognition of individuals' contributions and

---

18   TG2, Rai, 22 February 1999.

19   Bucchi 2017; on folk narratives of scientific discovery see also Brannigan 1981.

the ideal of the suppression of the self, supposedly essential to science [...] to insist on their ordinariness as a means to emphasize, by an effect of contrast, the extraordinariness of their work'.[20]

From the point of view of their role, the three presenters took a clear triangular disposition: on the two sides, two celebrities embodying qualities perfectly symmetric and equally admired and aspired to. The beauty of Laetitia Casta, who came from the glamorous world of hyper paid and hyper busy fashion models, and the intelligence of Renato Dulbecco, the Nobel Prize winner who until yesterday was inquiring into nature's best hidden secrets. Despite the extremely different professions, the two have in common this being special and 'different' from the general public watching at home – a difference which was underlined by the extremely elegant dress of the model and the highly formal suit worn by the scientist. Two stars, both apparently light years away from ordinary people.

Between them is Fazio, the main presenter of the show, inevitably taking up the role of the 'common person'; the spokesman for the desires and expectations of the public with whom he makes every effort to identify. Dressed less formally compared to them, Fazio shows great deference towards the two extraordinary personalities standing beside him.[21] 'At the age of 14, the same age when I and most of my fellows were trying to learn how to ride a Vespa, you invented an electronic seismograph. How did that spring to your mind?'. Fazio asked Dulbecco, emphasizing his own surprise. The distance between the presenter and the Nobel laureate is also underlined by the different attitudes that they have towards the French model. While Fazio is incarnating the stereotype of the common man mesmerized by the unreachable beauty of the star, Dulbecco shows the relative indifference typical of somebody who has quite different and more profound thoughts. 'Laetitia Casta is a big, rather complicated sea sponge', is the short description that the scientist offers to Fazio of the model, widely reprised by all news media during the following days. The presence of Dulbecco in this context takes the meaning of a 'descent' from high above by a figure otherwise unreachable by the 'common people':

> A man who has so strongly contributed to research, for example, of the polio vaccine, who at a certain stage in his life decides to take, at 85 years, five days of break, for me is a wonderful example for everybody.[22]

---

20   Gouyon 2018, 250.
21   On the Nobel Prize as a ritual expression of society's deference towards science, see Bucchi 2017; Bucchi 2018; on the sociological notion of deference see Goffman 1956.
22   Fazio to TV news Rai, 22 February 1999.

At the same time, however, from the presenter's interaction with the scientist during the Festival emerges how in the end, even in his detachment from mundane things that characterizes the public image of the scientist, Dulbecco remains a normal person, 'one of us'. 'He is just like us', Fazio keeps repeating during the TV program and at press conferences about the show. Dulbecco himself reinforced this interpretation of his involvement with the Festival:

> I am aware that some people say – but why does a scientist come here? Well first of all *the scientist is a person just like anybody else and I am here somehow to show you that I am interested in the same things you all are, that eventually there is nothing special about being a scientist.*[23]

Without at the same time failing to restate some of his own peculiarities as scientist:

> But during the first evening of the show, were you nervous just like all normal human beings? – No, you know, for me seeing the audience, talking to an audience is not a new experience because I often give talks...[24]

Both registers are summarized by his widely publicized statement on stage that he had 'come to the Festival for the sake of the experience', at the same time emphasizing his humility, naivety towards the show business and recalling a term that several commentators immediately associated with Galileo's widely known expression 'sensate esperienze'.[25] An ordinary person, still speaking like a scientist.

The Staging of a Genius

The tension between opposed 'discursive repertoires' has been identified by studies of scientific discourse as the main source of humor about science and among scientists. The humorous effect thereby often comes from juxtaposing the 'special' character of science to practices typical of everyday life; or from the short-circuiting between the informal repertoire that scientists adopt in 'private' contexts like the laboratory and the more formal repertoire of

---

23   TG1 Rai, 22 February 1999, italics by the author.
24   TG2 Rai, 24 February 1999.
25   G. Galilei, 'Lettera a Madama Cristina di Lorena', 1615, in Opere, a cura di F. Flora, Milano-Napoli, Ricciardi, 1953, 1013–1101.

scientific lectures and papers.[26] This aspect is highly visible in connection with the participation of Dulbecco in the Sanremo Festival, particularly when such participation is mocked by other TV programs. *Striscia la notizia*, a daily satirical news program, makes fun of Dulbecco's appearance by referring to a science issue that was quite salient in media and public discourse at the time: cloning.[27]

An actor resembling Dulbecco and introduced as his 'clone', visited Festival participants and guests who were mostly deceived and took him for the actual Dulbecco.[28] The humorous trick had a double symbolic value: on the one hand, according to a classic narrative model, a scientific theme of particular public salience and relevance like cloning was 'turned against' science. On the other hand, the alleged 'specialness' of Dulbecco was brought down to earth: he really is one of us, in the sense that anybody can replace him, if not in his expert capacity, at least in his public dimension. The satire focuses on the latter, precisely because it was what mattered in the public context. No one talked about Dulbecco's discoveries, nobody was interested in them. The only message was that Dulbecco was not present to represent himself, but rather science at large.

> Here, among true flowers that seem fake (and vice versa) the scientist Dulbecco says that Laetitia Casta is a great, complicated sponge while the girl does not resemble a sponge at all and does not seem too complicated. Thus science becomes a bit a ridiculous i.e. at everybody's reach.[29]

The short-circuiting between models and repertoires becomes complete when the satirical program, after the Festival was finished, broadcasted videos of the Festival rehearsals. This backstage exposure brought the intertwining of the two popular 'ideologies' of science to light.[30] Beside Casta and Dulbecco, Fazio had decided to bring on stage some representatives of 'common people' to occasionally introduce some songs and guests. During rehearsals, a woman from

---

26   Cfr. Mulkay and Gilbert 1982.
27   The issue of cloning had already become familiar to the Italian media and public, like in many other countries, following the announcement of the first cloned sheep 'Dolly' by a research team lead by scientist Ian Wilmut (1997). On the interaction between popular discourse and scientific discourse on themes like cloning see also Bucchi 2004.
28   It is no coincidence that the comedian imitating Dulbecco addressed a figure well known to the general public for her cooking books. Linking to or comparing with scientific activity is an often used strategy to present science as more 'human' and bringing it closer to common experience (Pinch 1992; Bucchi 2013).
29   *Il Corriere della Sera*, 27 February 1999.
30   On the concept of backstage with regard to social interaction see the classic Goffman (1959); in relation to science communication see Bucchi 1998.

these 'lay presenters' was unable to walk the long staircase leading to the stage. She asked 'to do like professor Dulbecco, and get on stage from the side door'. However, after a quick consultation with his staff, Fazio denied this possibility to her. Thus Dulbecco is like all of us, yes, but only up to a certain point. His 'specialness' guarantees him a privilege that it is not possible to extend to ordinary people without risking a collision between different roles and dignities. An exception could be made for him, but not for ordinary people.

Propaganda for Science or Halo Effect?

Overall, the main effect of the presence of Dulbecco at the Sanremo festival seems to be that of offering – more than scientific content – a sort of rhetorical resource ready for use, a resource that the different actors involved are not so interested to understand but rather to employ in other contexts. The presence of Dulbecco on the stage of Sanremo Festival created a sort of 'halo effect' by putting science on the agenda (although in a rhetorical, rather than in content-related sense), thereby activating themes and metaphors from the scientific domain. During the inaugural evening, for example, Fazio introduced the French model as 'a masterpiece of genetics', while the comedian Teocoli described Dulbecco as 'a magnet loaded with energy and enthusiasm'. During the final evening of the Festival, a comedian staged an imitation of another Nobel Prize winner, Rita Levi Montalcini, describing Fazio as 'Dulbecco's masterpiece: he is much more beautiful than Dolly the sheep'.

The Nobel laureate here acts as a sort of 'catalyst': science related issues which had emerged within public discourse during the preceding years (cloning, genetic modifications) were again referred to in the completely different media context. More broadly, *the mere presence* of Dulbecco on Sanremo stage evoked and embodied *Science*. This contributes to explain why so little relevance was given both to his own specific research activity and private life.[31] Another effect is related to Dulbecco's Nobel status. On repeated occasions, Fazio compared Dulbecco's appearances on the Sanremo theatre stage with his formal dress, as well as his participation in the distinctive ritual of the event of the Nobel ceremony: for example, by asking him about his feelings when receiving the Nobel medal from the hands of the King of Sweden.

---

31   This casting of Nobel laureates into a broader narrative of science – largely obliterating their individual specificities – is also partially found by Gouyon as a distinctive feature of BBC television productions involving Nobel laureates since the 1990s (Gouyon, 2018).

It could be argued that both the Sanremo Festival and the Nobel events share a strong ritual element, in both cases amplified by the mediatic dimension. Another element they share is the ritual of coronation, wherein a winner is recognized and rewarded, a type of ceremony symbolically centered on values of 'tradition and continuity'.[32] After years of crisis and decline, the Sanremo Festival tried to reaffirm its traditional ceremonial nature by connecting to the Nobel ritual through the presence of one of its protagonists. The Nobel Prizegiving ceremony can in fact be studied as a ritual 'through which the person is allotted a kind of sacredness that is displayed and confirmed by symbolic acts'. The central element of such ceremony is *deference* 'by which appreciation is conveyed to a recipient (...) or to something of which this recipient is taken as a symbol, extension, or agent'.[33] Thus, through the ceremony and the elaborate rituals of the Nobel week, deference is expressed towards the laureate, and through her or him, towards science at large.

Having a Nobel laureate on Sanremo stage, introducing singers and conferring the final Prize to the winner, partially transfers the deference to a ritual that in the past few years had seen its centrality in social and popular culture undermined. This defines a distinct and interesting way in which Nobel laureates 'demonstrate the social power of scientific celebrity' can become 'tradable cultural commodities': not just through their own individual scientific celebrity but dragging together with their presence at least some of the ritual elements – e.g. the ceremony and the royal touch consecrating the Prizewinner – that have contributed to make the Nobel Prize so visible and influential in shaping the public image of science in the twentieth century.[34] This element is emphasized by a scientist working in Dulbecco's laboratory, asked for an opinion about the laureate's suitability to present Sanremo: 'One like Dulbecco, he could well present also the Olympic Games'.[35]

The counterpart of deference is *demeanor*, i.e. 'the individual's behavior typically conveyed through deportment, dress, and bearing, which serves to express [...] that he is a person of certain qualities'.[36] Once a Nobel, one is a Nobel forever. Since the Nobel status confers not only recognition but moral authority, the behavior of laureates must be in line with these expectations not only during the very ritualized moments, but also after the Prize. Significantly, before the Festival, when Dulbecco's participation was announced, some of his

---

32   On media ceremonies see the classical Dayan and Katz 1992.
33   Goffman 1956, 477.
34   Fahy and Lewenstein 2014; Fahy 2018; Bucchi 2017; Bucchi 2018.
35   From an interview with Italian television, https://www.youtube.com/watch?v=9uBhqej
      V5cM (accessed February 26, 2019).
36   Goffman 1956, 489.

colleagues and commentators had expressed their concern that his involvement in Sanremo could 'contaminate' his Nobel status and even the status of the Prize and the public image of science at large. 'He obviously has time to waste' declared astrophysicist Margherita Hack, a scientist well known to the Italian public. 'He doesn't know in which trouble he is placing himself', said Nobel laureate in medicine Rita Levi Montalcini, and Nobel laureate in literature Dario Fo warned the scientist of possible risks as well. Dulbecco dismissed those concerns as part of an 'old attitude, typical of the scientist of the past who used to keep out of the rest of the world, in an ivory tower'.[37]

What about the public then? Was it actually 'propaganda for science' as Dulbecco had stated himself? A survey conducted on a representative sample of the general public immediately after the end of the 1999 Festival edition showed that the impact had been rather minor. Although the great majority of Italians, including those who had not watched the Festival on TV, were aware of Dulbeccos participation and identified him as a scientist, even his disciplinary affiliation remained confused. In fact, 22% of interviewees described him as a physicist or alchemist, and among those who had watched the whole Festival the percentage of those being unable to identify Dulbecco's scientific field was even higher than the corresponding percentage among non-viewers.[38]

The survey also provides hints of the opinions of interviewees on Dulbecco's participation to Sanremo. For most of them it was an important initiative 'because it demonstrated that science is made by persons like anybody else'. The presence of a world famous Nobel scientist to this popular show seems to have somehow contributed to 'desacralise' science and its key figures by showing their 'human side'. It is no coincidence that such an opinion is expressed more frequently by those who express great trust in science: confidence in science coincides with the need to emphasize its normality as an antidote to suspicions and concerns that often emerge with regard to science related issues such as GMOs, genetic editing, embryo stem cell research and cloning.[39] Adversely, those who have less trust in science not only tend to underplay the relevance of Dulbecco's participation to Sanremo in terms of public understanding of science, but also tend to share more frequently critical

---

37 All quotations are from an interview with Italian television https://www.youtube.com/watch?v=9uBhqejV5cM (accessed February 26, 2019).

38 The sample included 739 subjects aged over 15 and it was designed in order to be representative of the Italian population by gender, age, and area of residence. For a more detailed analysis of the survey results see Bucchi and Neresini 2000.

39 On general features and trends of public perception of science in Italy, see for example Bucchi and Saracino 2014. On public attitudes to biotechnologies, see Bucchi and Neresini 2002; Bucchi and Neresini 2004.

judgements like 'science is too serious as an enterprise to mix it with Sanremo Festival'.

Overall, thus, more than having actually contributed to the spread of scientific content and stimulating interest for science, as Dulbecco had initially hoped, the presence of a Nobel laureate in a media event as visible as the Sanremo Festival seems to have unfolded along two main communicative dimensions. The first dimension is that of the aforementioned dynamic of 'prestige transfer'. After a few editions which had not been particularly successful, the Festival and its new presenter Fabio Fazio brought a Nobel laureate on stage as part of a 'requalification strategy'. This strategy put at the center the contamination and mix of genres and formats and tries to appropriate not just the visibility, but also the status of a scientist 'crowned' at the highest level to revitalize and reconfirm its own status of media ritual. The second dimension unfolded via the presence of a Nobel prizewinner on stage at the very visible media event of the Sanremo Festival. This significantly contributed to establishing on the public agenda – as well as to personifying – the growing relevance of science and science related issues in public discourse.

Bibliography

Anselmi, A. 2009. *Festival di Sanremo*. Modena: Panini.

Beltrame, L. 2007. 'Ipse Dixit. I premi Nobel come argomento di autorità nella comunicazione pubblica della scienza'. *Studi di Sociologia* 1: 77–98.

Brannigan, A. 1981. *The Social Basis of Scientific Discoveries*. Cambridge: Cambridge University Press.

Bucchi, M. 1998. *Science and the Media*. London and New York: Routledge.

Bucchi, M. 2004. *Science in Society: An Introduction to Social Studies of Science*. London: Routledge.

Bucchi, M. 2004b. 'Can Genetics Help Us Rethink Communication? Public Communication of Science as a 'Double Helix''. *New Genetics and Society* 23(3): 269–283.

Bucchi, M. 2013. *Il pollo di Newton. La scienza in cucina*. Parma: Guanda.

Bucchi, M. 2015. 'Norms, competition and visibility in contemporary science: The legacy of Robert K. Merton'. *Journal of Classical Sociology* 15(3): 233–252.

Bucchi, M. 2017. *Come vincere un Nobel. L'immagine pubblica della scienza e il suo premio più famoso*. Torino: Einaudi (English edition forthcoming in 2019, *Geniuses, Heroes and Saints. The Nobel Prize and the Public Image of Science*. Cambridge: MIT Press.).

Bucchi, M. 2018. '"The winner takes it all?" Nobel laureates and the public image of science', *Public Understanding of Science*, 27(4): 390–396.

Bucchi, M. and Neresini, F. 2000. 'Un Nobel a Sanremo (ma la scienza rimane sconosciuta)'. *Problemi dell'informazione* 2: 233–250.

Bucchi, M. and Neresini, F. 2002. 'Biotech Remains Unloved by the More Informed'. *Nature* 416: 261.

Bucchi, M. and Neresini, F. 2004. 'Why Are People Hostile to Biotechnologies?'. *Science*: 1749.

Bucchi, M. and Saracino, B. 2014. 'Gli italiani, la scienza e le tecnologie: dieci tendenze che hanno segnato il rapporto tra cittadini e scienza, 2002–2013'. In *Annuario Scienza e Società 2014. Dieci anni di scienza nella società*, edited by M. Bucchi and B. Saracino, 15–54. Bologna: Il Mulino.

Bucchi, M. and Trench, B. 2014. 'Science communication research: themes and challenges'. In *Handbook of Public Communication of Science and Technology*, edited by M. Bucchi and B. Trench, 1–13. London and New York: Routledge.

Dayan, D. and Katz, E. 1992 *Media Events*, Harvard University Press, Cambridge, MA.

Fahy, D. 2018. 'The laureate as celebrity genius: How Scientific American's John Horgan profiled Nobel Prize winners'. *Public Understanding of Science* 27(4): 433–445.

Fahy, D. and Lewenstein, B. 2014. 'Scientists in popular culture'. In *Handbook of Public Communication of Science and Technology*, edited by M. Bucchi and B. Trench, 83–96. London and New York: Routledge.

Goodel, R. 1997. *The Visible Scientists*. Boston: Little Brown.

Goffman, E. 1956. 'The Nature of Deference and Demeanor'. *American Anthropologist* 58(3): 473–502.

Goffman, E. 1959. *The Presentation of Self in Everyday Life*. New York: Doubleday.

Gouyon 2018. 'From engaged citizen to lone hero: Nobel Prize laureates on British television, 1962–2004'. *Public Understanding of Science* 27(4): 446–457.

Merton, R.K. 1973. *The Matthew Effect in Science*, repr. in *The Sociology of Science. Theoretical and Empirical Investigations*. Chicago: University of Chicago Press.

Mulkay, M. and Gilbert, N. 1982. 'Joking Apart: Some Recommendations concerning the Social Study of Science', *Social Studies of Science*, 12: 585–614.

Pinch, T. 1992. Opening Black Boxes: Sciences, Technology and Society, in 'Social Studies of Science', 22, 3: 487–510.

Pratt, D. 2012. *Nobel Wisdom: The 1000 Wisest Things Ever Said*. London: JR Books Ltd.

Zuckerman, H. 1996 [1977]. *Scientific Elite: Nobel Laureates in the United States*. New Brunswick, NJ: Transactions.

CHAPTER 9

Nobel Prize Awarded Discoveries and Commercialization: The Role of the Laureates

Katarina Nordqvist and Pauline Mattsson

The Nobel Prize was built from the industrial empire that Alfred Nobel created in the second half of the nineteenth century. His businesses were based on several patents. In 1864 he patented the detonator, which made it possible to control the explosive substance nitro-glycerine, enabling it to become a commercial product. Nobel's strategy was to get onto the market as quickly as possible by establishing companies and factories in several countries. In 1867 he invented dynamite, a safer explosive based on nitro-glycerine. Patents for various types of dynamite, including blasting gelatine, became major assets in his businesses. By his death in 1896, Alfred Nobel had more than 300 patents registered to his name, and some 90 factories in about 20 countries had arisen from companies started by Nobel.[1]

In his will, he announced that the greater part of his estate – valued at 31 million Swedish kronor at the time – would be used to establish a prize. The returns on this capital have since then been used for the awarding of Nobel Prizes. Alfred Nobel stated in his will that prizes shall be awarded to those who 'have conferred the greatest benefit to mankind' in the fields of physics, chemistry, physiology or medicine, literature, and work to promote peace. Since the first Nobel Prizes were awarded in 1901, the Prize-awarding institutions have been faced with the challenge to relate to the phrase 'greatest benefit to mankind' when selecting the Laureate(s). Nobel didn't give an interpretation of the phrase, and it is therefore impossible to know exactly what his intentions had been. A book about Alfred Nobel published by the Nobel Foundation in 1925 presents some suggestions of what Nobel may have had in mind.[2] One witness says that Nobel had declared on various occasions that he primarily would like to benefit scientists, since they often have difficulties monetizing their results, from which others benefit. Contemporary accounts also state that he viewed the will solely as showing the general direction of his intentions, and that he trusted the Nobel Prize-awarding institutions to develop instructions

---

1　Frängsmyr 2008; Larsson 2008.
2　Nobelstiftelsens styrelse 1925.

and award prizes in line with his vision. Together with the statutes of the Nobel Foundation, which were officially approved by the Swedish Government on June 29, 1900, the will constitutes the basis on which the Prize-awarding institutions carry out their work. In 1926, Jöns Johansson, then Chairman of the Medical Nobel Committee, wrote a memorandum document for the work of selecting the Nobel prize in Physiology or Medicine.[3] When discussing the phrase 'the greatest benefit to mankind', Johansson writes that the discovery could be awarded in any medical field and without any regard to the monetary aspects.[4]

Most Nobel Prizes have been awarded for breakthroughs in various research fields. A 'breakthrough' can be defined as a discovery that disturbs previous understanding in a fundamental manner, opening up new scientific and/or technological avenues.[5] Breakthroughs are first published as scientific papers, which become a primary source for the dissemination of knowledge. Research and innovation have long been seen as major drivers for forming prosperous societies and Alfred Nobel is a great example of an inventor who successfully brought his inventions to the (global) market. During the 20th century, especially after the Second World War, there was a firm belief among governments that research and development form the cornerstone for a thriving and sustainable society. Vast resources were invested into research and development (R&D), with the expectation of a return on investment. Returns may be in the form of a more educated and skilled workforce, increased knowledge based on scientific discoveries and breakthroughs, a flow of brilliant ideas and inventions that could be commercialized, thriving start-ups and well-established companies, and a healthier population. Today, it is well established that research and development are important foundations for the development of a sound economy and prosperous society,[6] and many countries are investing significantly in R&D.[7] One of the cornerstones of the knowledge-based economy is the production of novel ideas and scientific breakthroughs.

In this chapter we focus on biomedical breakthroughs for which the Nobel Prize in Physiology or Medicine has been awarded. Many of these breakthroughs have proven to be indisputable factors in the improvement of human health and the basis of innovations and industrial development. Examples

---

3 Johansson 1926.
4 (In Swedish) '...han betraktade det också blott såsom ett dokument, som angav den riktning, i vilken han ville att de där givna bestämmelserna skulle vidare utformas för att *göra mänskligheten den största nyttan*'; *Alfred Nobel och hans släkt*, 256.
5 Tushman and Anderson 1986; Chai 2014.
6 Romer 1990; Nelson 1996; Mokyr 2003.
7 National Science Board 2018.

include the discovery of insulin and penicillin, the generation of monoclonal antibodies, and the development of computer-assisted tomography.[8] But how have these breakthroughs translated into something useful for society? Which are the diffusion mechanisms of breakthroughs? Which actors are involved in this process? These questions have attracted scholars from many disciplines and their answers are found in research on creativity, research production, innovation systems and entrepreneurship. Broadly, this research into the conduct of science can be divided into the levels of individuals, institutions and nations, although all levels are highly interconnected. Here we focus on the individual researcher, more specifically on the role of the Laureates, in the early process of translating their discoveries into useful innovation. Even though scientific research has generally become more collaborative,[9] earlier studies highlighted the importance of the individual researcher in the translation of research into innovations. The idea is that knowledge transfer is mainly person-embodied, involving personal contacts, movements, and participation in national and international networks.[10] Furthermore, previous studies have shown that the distribution of output is strongly skewed among scientists,[11] highlighting the importance of studying the scientific elite.

In this chapter, we will investigate how Nobel Prize awarded discoveries have come into wider use. More specifically, we examine how Laureates have been involved in the innovation and diffusion processes by which their results were commercialized. We attempt to determine whether the intention of Alfred Nobel's will – to serve 'the greatest benefit to mankind' – has been satisfied. We will focus on the breakthrough discoveries awarded the Nobel Prize in Physiology or Medicine between 1978 and 2013 and investigate the subsequent activities of the Nobel Laureates in the translation and commercialization of their discoveries. This study looks at the Laureates' entire career and focuses on the dissemination of knowledge and the extent to which the Nobel Laureates were involved in applying for patents, starting spin-offs and consulting or even collaborating with industry.

Our initial hypothesis was that new knowledge that is eventually awarded the Nobel Prize is embedded in the Nobel Laureates' 'intellectual human capital'. Earlier literature has shown that the knowledge behind breakthrough discoveries is of a tacit character that can only be transmitted through

---

8   Thompson 2012.
9   Wuchty et al. 2007.
10   Gibbons and Johnston 1974; Bruneel et al. 2010.
11   de Solla Price 1963; Merton 1968; Zuckerman 1967, 1970, 1977.

personal interaction.[12] This suggests that the Laureates would be deeply involved in translating their discoveries into wider use, including commercial
activities. If this theory/prediction holds, it is contrary to what we believe to be
Alfred Nobel's intentions of the Prize: to award it to those scientists who have
made a high-impact discovery, but with few possibilities to monetize it.

Methods

We have studied the biomedical discoveries, and the 83 Laureates awarded
the Nobel Prize in Physiology or Medicine between 1978 and 2013. We chose
this time period since data (such as publications and patents) are more readily
available for this period, and it is possible to find information about industrial
involvement. We collected information about all 83 Laureates' publications using the *Web of Science*.[13] To make sure that we had included all publications of
Nobel Laureates and excluded publications by authors with the same names,
we compared the collected WoS publications with CVs and biographies,
checked the authors' addresses, and read the abstracts. To determine whether
the Laureates had carried out research with industrial partners, we searched
for company names in the address field. We then classified any companies thus
found as 'multinational companies' (MNCs), which we defined as companies
with more than 500 employees; 'small and medium enterprises' (SMEs), defined as companies with less than 500 employees; or 'start-ups' defined as companies that the Laureates had been involved in starting.

We used both USPTO and Espacenet to search for patents.[14] Applications
for patents and patents that had been granted were identified by matching
the name of the Laureate with the name of the inventor and using the address from which the application had been filed and the content of the patent
to verify that the patent was indeed linked to a Laureate. Again, we searched
manually for company names in the applicant's field, and classified the companies thus found as MNCs, SMEs, or start-ups. Universities and research institutes (such as the Whitehead Biomedical Institute, Max Planck Gesellschaft,
the French National Centre for Scientific Research) were also included. Information regarding start-ups was collected from several online databases
(Bloomberg Business, Newswire, NNDP, Who's Who), Laureates' biographies,

---

12   Murray 2004.
13   www.webofknowledge.com (accessed February 26, 2019).
14   http://www.uspto.gov/patents-application-process/search-patents   and   http://world-
      wide.espacenet.com/ (accessed February 26, 2019).

CVs, and internet searches using a combination of the Laureate's name and the search terms *spin-off* and/or *founder*. Information collected in this way was verified by cross referencing with annual reports and websites of the companies, using Internet Archive.

The Value of Scientific Publications

For scientists, publishing implies following the norms of communism[15] in that scientists' research results are made available to the rest of the scientific community. Publications are, therefore, the primary information source for new knowledge. Counting publications and citations thereof has become a tool to measure scientific productivity, and are important criteria to determine eligibility for funding and promotion. This gives further incentives to publish.[16] As early as 1968, Eugene Garfield, founder of the Science Citation Index (SCI), used numbers of citations to predict who would be awarded the Nobel Prizes in 1969. He used the SCI database to identify the fifty most cited authors of 1967. Two of the 1969 Nobel Laureates, Derek H.R. Barton and Murray Gell-Mann, appeared on the list.[17] Since 2002, citations have been used by Thomson Reuters to identify its 'Citation Laureates' to predict Nobel Prize Laureates.

We have investigated the publication activity of the Nobel Laureates selected in this study. Figure 9.1 presents the h-index and the highest cited paper of each of the Laureates during their career. The h-index differs considerably between Laureates, with extreme values of 8 and 182, with a median value of 73. Also, the numbers of citations for the highest cited paper varies much, from around 400 to over 17,000 citations.

It is important, however, to remember the limitations of using citations to identify high-quality research, and that different scientific fields have different citation patterns. In very specialized fields the citation rates will be low, since the numbers of active researchers in such fields are low. One example of this is developmental biologist John Gurdon, who was awarded the Nobel Prize in 2012. He had a relatively low h-index and was not listed by Thomson Reuters in their predictions for 2012. The list did, however, include Shinya Yamanaka, who shared the Prize with Gurdon.[18] In addition, certain fields are more

---

15   Merton 1942.
16   Cronin and Sugimoto 2014.
17   Garfield and Malin 1968; Garfield 1970.
18   http://images.info.science.thomsonreuters.biz/Web/ThomsonReutersScience/ {00437ee8-8b0b-4872-bbd8-1303ff321e06}_CitationLaureates_Methodology_092016_002 .pdf (accessed February 26, 2019).

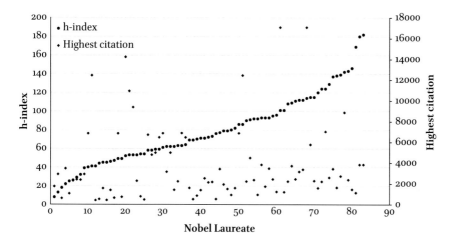

FIGURE 9.1   h-index and highest number of citations for Laureates awarded the Nobel Prize in Physiology or Medicine between 1978 and 2013

'dependent' on other fields. For example, clinical medicine draws heavily on basic science, but not vice versa. In consequence, papers in basic medicine are cited 3–5 times more often than those in clinical medicine.[19] Studies based on citation data using Nobel Prizes in chemistry and physics from 1901 to 2007 suggest that it has become more difficult to use bibliometrics to make predictions because of changes in the size and organization of fields, and due to an implicit hierarchy in the most legitimate topics within the discipline, and among the scientists selected for the Nobel Prize.[20]

The fields in which the Nobel Prizes are awarded can be divided into subfields. As early as 1926, when Johansson described the work of the Nobel Committee, the field of physiology and medicine was subdivided into six groups.[21] At the centennial celebration of the Nobel Prize in 2001, Jan Lindsten and Nils Ringertz (both of whom have been members of the Nobel Committee), grouped the Prizes in Physiology or Medicine into eighteen different headings.[22] Johansson created subgroups in 1926 to enable the Nobel Committee to group incoming nominations, while the subgroups defined in 2001 indicated the nature of the Nobel Prizes awarded during the previous 100 years. It is, however, interesting to note that the number of subfields is higher in 2001 than in 1926 (Table 9.1), which probably reflects the development of medical

---

19   Narin et al. 1976; Folly et al. 1981.
20   Gingras and Wallace 2010.
21   Johansson 1926.
22   Lindsten and Ringertz 2001.

TABLE 9.1   Subgrouping of Nobel Prizes in Physiology or Medicine, in 1926 by J.E Johansson
and in 2001 by J. Lindsten and N. Ringertz (the numbers in parentheses are the
years in which a Nobel Prize was awarded in this subfield).

1926	2001
I. Anatomy and histology (Anatomi och histologi)	Infectious agents and insecticides (1902, 1905, 1907, 1928, 1948, 1951, 1954, 1976, 1997)
II. Biology in general, Physiology, Physiological Chemistry, Pharmacology (Allmän biologi, fysiologi, fysiologisk kemi, läkemedelslära)	Immunology (1901, 1908, 1913, 1919, 1930, 1960, 1972, 1980, 1984, 1987, 1996)
III. Pathology and Pathological Anatomy (Patologi och patologisk anatomi)	Chemotherapy/drug development (1939, 1945, 1952, 1957, 1988)
IV. Medicine, Surgery, Therapy (Medicin, kirurgi, terapi)	Phototherapy and fever treatment (1903, 1927)
V. Bacteriology, Aetiology, Hygiene (Bakteriologi, etiologi, hygien)	Cancer (1926, 1966, 1975, 1989)
VI. Immunology (Immunitetslära)	Classical genetics (1933, 1946, 1983)
	Cell Biology (1974, 1986, 1999)
	Developmental Biology (1935, 1995)
	Molecular biology/genetics (1910, 1958, 1959, 1962, 1965, 1968, 1969, 1978, 1993)
	Intermediary metabolism (1922, 1931, 1937, 1947, 1953, 1955, 1964, 1982, 1985, 1992, 1994)
	Hormones (1909, 1923, 1947, 1950, 1971, 1998)
	Vitamins (1929, 1934, 1943)
	Digestion, circulation and respiration (1904, 1920, 1924, 1938, 1956)
	Neurobiology (1906, 1932, 1936, 1944, 1949, 1957, 1963, 1970, 1977, 1981, 1991, 2000)
	Surgery (1949, 1990)
	Sensory physiology (1911, 1914, 1961, 1967, 1981)
	Behavioral sciences (1973)
	Diagnostic methods (1979)

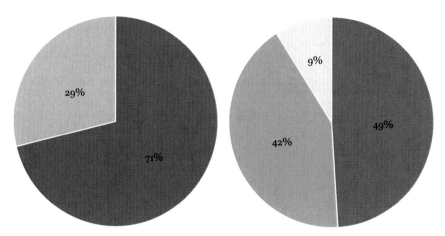

FIGURE 9.2   (A) While 71% of the Nobel Laureates applied for patents, 29% did not (B) Nobel
Laureates who have applied for patents together with only academic co-
applicants (49%), with industry co-applicants (42%), Laureates who have applied
while working for a company (9%).

research. In the period 1901–2000, this was characterised by an immense ac-
cumulation of knowledge due to the advancement of research, and diversifica-
tion and specialization into more narrowly defined fields.

The Commercialization of Nobel Prize Awarded Discoveries

Patenting is often the first step in the commercialization of biomedical research and possibly the most frequently used measure of scientists' involvement in this process. Despite its popularity as a measure of knowledge transfer, patenting is a rather minor activity among researchers. Agrawal and
Henderson (2002) found that 10–20% of MIT engineering faculty submit a patent application in any given year. Azoulay et al. (2007) focused on life-science
researchers and found that 12% of basic faculty and 3% of clinical faculty were
patent holders. Focusing on a sample of superstar scientists in the life sciences,
Azoulay et al. (2012) showed that about 60% have taken at least one patent
during their research career. This suggests that elite scientists act differently
than the general scientific population when it comes to patenting.

We have investigated the patent activity of the Nobel Laureates selected in
this study. Fifty-nine of the 83 Laureates (71%) have applied for a patent at
least once during their career (Figure 9.2A). Forty-nine percent of the Laureates who appear as inventors of a discovery for which a patent is applied took

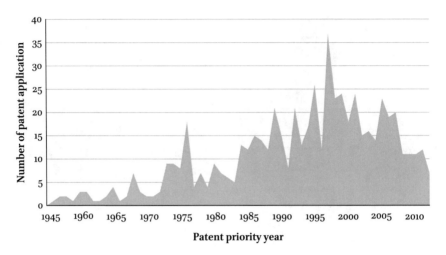

FIGURE 9.3 Patent applications by Nobel Laureates over time

all their patents together with a university or institute, while 42% collaborated with a company in their patent applications at least once (Figure 9.2B).

We conclude that Laureates have a higher propensity to patent than the general scientific population. We proceeded to investigate the patent activity of Laureates over time. Figure 9.3 shows that the total number of patent applications increased until the end of the 1990s and has been decreasing since then. This agrees with previous results from life-science faculty.[23] However, we see a downturn after 2000. This is related to the end of the human genome project that was responsible for the unprecedented growth in large-scale sequencing in the 1990s but also new guidelines, that prevented patenting of a sequence or partial sequence of a gene, within both the European Patent Office as well as the US Patent and Trademark Office (USPTO).

Part of the reason for the increase in patenting is the establishment of technology transfer offices (TTOs) at universities first in the US but then also in European countries, where most of the Laureates have been active. These offices arose as a consequence of the Bayh-Dole Act (effective in 1980), which changed the ownership of inventions that arose from work with governmental funding to the university, small business, or non-profit institution at which the work had been carried out. Other factors that contributed to the increase include an increase in interest in commercialization among researchers, and the large numbers of patents granted for gene sequences, as a result of the Human Genome Project. However, the Supreme Court in the US declared in 2013 that

---

23   Azoulay et al. 2007.

naturally occurring DNA sequences are not eligible for patents. Also, licensing through TTOs has long been central to university and government efforts to commercialize research.[24]

While patenting is an important channel for commercializing publicly funded research, other channels are available, and appear to be increasing in importance.[25] Earlier studies have shown that research productivity is positively correlated with involvement with industrial partners.[26] In contrast, other studies have shown that industrial collaboration has detrimental effects on research productivity.[27] Co-publication has been a frequently used metric to assess academic collaboration with industry.[28] Link et al. (2006) studied a population of 'normal' scientists and found that 28% have co-authored with an industrial partner. Zucker and Darby (2007) showed that almost 70% of highly cited researchers write at least one article with at least one industrial employee, and 10% of all articles written by these researchers can be linked to a company. They further identified these companies and showed that they are mainly start-ups created around the star scientist.[29]

We identified and analysed joint publications between Nobel Laureates and industrial actors. The Laureates collaborated with industry to a high degree. Seventy-nine percent of the Laureates had co-authored at least one publication with a company. The frequency increased with time, and the number of co-publications with industry was twice as high in the 1990s as it had been in the 1970s. The number of articles co-published with multinational companies (MNCS) is more than twice as many as the number published with small and medium enterprises (SMEs) (Figure 9.4). Even though there is a significant difference between the total numbers of articles co-published with the different categories of industrial actor (MNC, SME, start-up), the total number of MNCs, SMEs and start-up companies are similar (96, 103 and 97). Sixty-one Nobel Laureates have published at least once with an MNC, 47 with SMEs and 14 with their own start-ups. The GlaxoSmithKline group has co-authored most with Laureates, appearing in 18 articles. Other common collaborating companies are Genentech and Hoffmann-La Roche. We conclude that joint projects between the Laureates and industrial partners are common. Not all collaborations are finalized as joint publications, and this means that the metric underestimates the degree of collaboration with industry.

---

24   OECD 2013.
25   Perkmann 2013; OECD 2013.
26   Mansfield 1995; Van Looy et al. 2006.
27   Evans 2010; Slaughter and Leslie 2001; Behrens and Gray 2001.
28   Sorenson and Fleming 2004; Lundberg et al. 2006; Tijssen 2006.
29   Zucker et al. 2002.

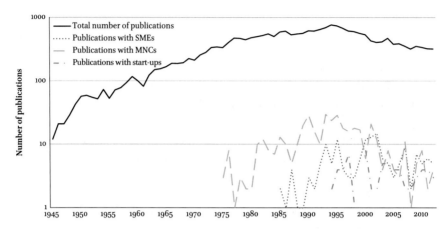

FIGURE 9.4   Total number of publications and with industry: Co-publication over time. The
             year of publication is depicted on the x-axis. The total number of publications,
             extracted by Web of Science (WoS), made by Laureates is shown on the
             y-axis. From 1973 WoS records addresses, making it possible to identify
             industry co-publications

The founding of start-up companies also indicates involvement in industrial
activities. Star scientists have had a major impact on the commercialization
of biotechnology through affiliations or links with new biotech companies,[30]
and academics with a high frequency of publication are more frequently involved in start-ups.[31] These collaborations have positive effects on the success
of a company. Higgins et al. (2011) used the status signal theory to study the
impact that the affiliation of Nobel Laureates with a technology-based firm in
an emerging industry has on an initial public offering (IPO). Companies with
which a Laureate was affiliated realized greater IPO proceeds than companies
without a Laureate. This effect is significant only in the early stage of the life of a
company and disappears when companies become more mature. The authors
suggest that having a Nobel Laureate affiliated with a company as it makes its
IPO provides a signal of the quality of the company to potential investors. The
importance of this signal diminishes when other metrics of the quality of the
company (such as the number of patent applications filed and the establishment of clinical trials) become available. Previous studies have suggested that
the knowledge that underlies the inventions on which such companies are
based tends to be of tacit character, and that it is paramount that the founder

30   Zucker and Darby 1996.
31   Perkmann et al. 2011.

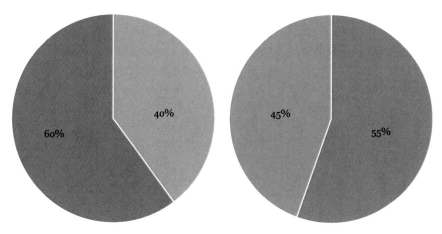

FIGURE 9.5   (a) Nobel Laureates involved in starting a company (40%) or not (60%), and (b) Nobel Laureates appointed to a scientific advisory board (55%) or not (45%)

is involved in further technology development.[32] Academic founders not only contribute tacit knowledge to the company, but also provide network ties that are particularly rich in research knowledge and social capital.[33]

Thirty-three of the Laureates studied here (40%, Figure 9.5) had participated in starting a company and fifty-five companies were identified in which a Laureate had been involved. Fourteen Laureates had been involved in starting more than one company. Most start-up companies were started after 1995. Previous studies of start-ups in which the academic founder was present[34] have shown that the survival rate of the start-up companies is high, and our results confirm this: only four out of 55 underwent liquidation. We investigated whether the Laureates who were involved in a company had left academia in order to become affiliated with the business full-time, in order to help the company grow. Few of the Laureates had an address linked to industry, and only one Laureate left academia to work in his own start-up company as a full-time employee. Thus, nearly all of the star scientists remain in academia, performing research instead of building business.

Most of the Laureates who become involved in a start-up company are elected to the board of directors, often in a scientific advisory role. Perkmann and Walsh (2008) distinguish between opportunity-driven, commerce-driven, and research-driven consulting, and show that consulting has only a limited

---

32   Owe 2002; Thursby 2004.
33   Murray 2004; Löfsten 2005.
34   Nekar 2003.

impact in pushing academic research into a more 'applied' direction. They argue that consulting is positively associated with academics' research productivity for research-driven and, to a lesser extent, commerce-driven consulting, while involvement in opportunity-driven consulting has a negative impact. We have examined the engagement of Nobel Laureates with industry in the form of membership of scientific advisory boards (SABs). Forty-six of the Laureates (55%) participated at least once in an SAB during their career (Figure 9.4B). Consulting and SAB involvement are more common in SMEs (41 Nobel Laureates) than in MNCs (25 Nobel Laureates).

The Translation of Nobel Prize Awarded Discoveries into Wider Use

Discoveries awarded the Nobel Prize are not only invaluable sources of new knowledge for other researchers to build on: many have been developed directly or indirectly into a product or process of importance for mankind. This is true for the Nobel Prize in Physiology or Medicine, where many discoveries have been the foundation for novel preventions, diagnostics and treatments.[35]

One example is the discovery of the principle for production of monoclonal antibodies by César Milstein and Georges Köhler (awarded the Nobel Prize in 1984). This technology, the hybridoma technology, was initially used to produce specific antibodies and early on became very important diagnostic tools for disease monitoring as well as for blood and tissue typing. It was subsequently developed and used in the development of drugs and helped to improve the treatment of over fifty diseases. Some of the major applications of these drugs are in treating various cancers and inflammatory and autoimmune disorders.[36] Milstein and Köhler were not granted a patent for the hybridoma technology,[37] but Milstein was highly involved in many of the projects that followed the discovery, working to increase and refine the areas of use of monoclonal antibodies for both diagnostics and therapeutics. He and his colleagues at the MRC Laboratory of Molecular Biology, Cambridge, UK, played an important part in demonstrating and introducing the hybridoma technique to other scientists, including sending samples to the research community, following the key publication by Köhler and Milstein in Nature in 1975.[38]

---

35   Thomson 2012.
36   http://www.whatisbiotechnology.org/science/mabs (accessed February 26, 2019).
37   de Chadarevian 2011.
38   Marks 2015.

A second example of the successful translation is the discovery by James Black, Gertrude Elion and George Hitchings of important principles for drug treatment. They shared the Nobel Prize in Physiology or Medicine in 1988 for their work using a rational approach in drug development, based on an understanding of basic biochemical and physiological processes. These Laureates are among few who worked in industry when they made their breakthrough discoveries. The original idea of Elion and Hitchings was to look for differences in nucleic acid metabolism between normal and cancer cells. Based on their research on the bacterium *Lactobacillus casei*, they developed substances that can block nucleic acid synthesis in cancer cells, and these were used in clinical trials in patients to treat leukemia. In short, they carried out basic research while employed within industry, with a strong focus on solving a medical problem – to treat cancer. This was followed by the normal process for developing a drug, including clinical trials and approval of the drugs for wider use, benefiting mankind.

Conclusion

We present here investigations into Nobel Laureates and their breakthrough discoveries that have been judged by the Nobel Committee to 'benefit mankind'. These discoveries have had a major impact on our understanding of biological and medical processes, and many have also been the basis for novel prevention, diagnostics and treatment. Many have thus found widespread use in society. We have used databases (*Web of Science*, USPTO, Espacenet, Bloomberg Business, Newswire, NNDP, Who's Who), the biographies and CVs of Laureates, and internet searches to select the past 35 years' Nobel Prizes, and to identify publications, patent applications and industry activities of the 83 Laureates who were awarded the Nobel Prize during this period. The Nobel Laureates were working in a wide variety of subfields, and their discoveries within the domain of physiology and medicine are diverse, from clinical breakthroughs, such as organ transplantation, to basic mechanisms, such as telomere function.

Publications are the primary information source for new knowledge. Counting publications and citations thereof has become a tool to measure scientific productivity, including high-impact research. Many have tried to come up with prediction models when it comes to who will be awarded the Nobel Prize. Judged by the large differences in both h-index between Laureates but also by the different citation rates of the Nobel prize awarded research it makes it difficult to find a common pattern between the different breakthrough discoveries.

In addition, one can only speculate how the classification of different subfields and the structure of science will look like in decades from now.

The behaviour of most of the 83 Nobel Laureates selected for this study was similar to the behaviour of previously studied 'star scientists' with respect to frequency of commercialization and collaborations with industry, measured through co-authorships, patent applications and start-up companies. Overall, patent activity was high, with 71% of the Laureates having made at least one patent application. Industry activities are also high, with 40% of the Laureates being involved in starting a company and 55% being active on scientific advisory boards in companies. Also, 79% have made at least one co-publication with an industrial partner.

Three groups of Laureates can be identified, one with high commercial activity (approx. 30% of the Laureates), one with lower commercial activity (approx. 25% of the Laureates), and one with almost no commercial activity (approx. 45% of the Laureates). It is also clear that more recent Laureates are more commercially active than older Laureates, taking more patents and being more involved in start-ups, which is consistent with a rise in commercial activities by academics in general since the 1980s.[39] Most Laureates, however, remain in academia, which suggest a strong desire to continue doing research after being awarded the Nobel Prize. To understand the role of the Laureates in translating breakthrough discoveries into innovations, it is also important to investigate their initial view on science and their major driving forces for conducting research. The biographies reveal that the Laureates are driven mainly by curiosity, to answer a specific question primarily because a certain topic is of interest to them. The topic may be a medical need or simply a quest to find out how a certain biological process works.

Many of the Prize-awarded discoveries drove a paradigm shift, and these normally take time to be broadly accepted. This may be the reason that few breakthrough discoveries have been translated directly into innovations by the Laureates. Further, it may take many years, and may require the involvement of many actors and institutions, before an initial discovery is developed into a final innovation that is widely used in science (such as the patch-clamp technique), or in society (such as the monoclonal antibodies used to treat diseases). A few Laureates worked within or in close collaboration with industrial partners, and in such cases the discoveries have been directly translated in a company setting. Example of this include the development of H_2 receptor antagonists against peptic ulcer, the use of 6-mercaptopurine against leukemia, and the use of pyrimethamine against malaria. However, in most cases,

---

39   Azoulay et al. 2007.

collaboration with industry takes place at a rather late stage of the Laureates' careers, and our results suggest that it is mainly other actors who drive the development and commercialization of Nobel-awarded discoveries.

In conclusion, about half of the Laureates have been actively involved in the very early stages of commercialization. The quantitative analysis presented here does not include in-depth interviews with Laureates. These would give deeper understanding of the incentives and the roles played by Nobel Laureates in the translation and commercialization of their discoveries. Such interviews would give a broader and more comprehensive view of the early phases of innovation pathways of high-impact research. The innovation pathways of specific discoveries should also be investigated, and the actors and institutions involved identified and their specific roles clarified, to obtain a deeper understanding of the process.

It is possible to view every discovery that has been awarded a Nobel Prize in Physiology or Medicine and ask if this is what Nobel had in mind. Has the selection of discoveries been in line with Nobel's will? It is, of course, impossible to know since the will is short and gives only few guidelines about how to select the Nobel Prize Laureates. It is clear that the Nobel Prizes have highlighted many important discoveries, but there are many more discoveries that have not been awarded, some of which can be found in the nomination archive/database.[40] Nobel had intended to benefit scientists, since they usually have difficulties monetizing their results, from which others benefit. The work presented here suggests that this is indeed the case: most Laureates have not focused on monetizing their results. Most of the Laureates investigated in this study have made discoveries that have benefited mankind. After making their discoveries, a majority of the Laureates continued in research and building further knowledge rather than focusing on commercialization and building a business.

Acknowledgements

This study was undertaken as part of the project 'Research for the benefit of mankind – Lessons learned from the Nobel Prizes in Medicine'. We gratefully acknowledge the financial support of the Swedish Research Council (grant B0210101). We thank Stephanie Wood, Åsa Michelgård Palmquist, Swati Ravi, Michael Hezel and Ulf Larsson for essential help and valuable comments.

---

40   https://www.nobelprize.org/nomination/archive/ (accessed February 26, 2019).

Bibliography

Agrawal, A. and Henderson, R. 2002. 'Putting Patents in Context: Exploring Knowledge Transfer from MIT'. *Management Science* 48(1): 44–60.

Azoulay, P.; Graff Zivin, J.S.; Sampat, B.N. 2012. 'The Diffusion of Scientific Knowledge across Time and Space Evidence from Professional Transitions for the Superstars of Medicine'. In *The Rate of Direction of Inventive Activity*, edited by J. Lerner and S. Stern, 107–155. Chicago and London: University of Chicago Press.

Azoulay, P.; Michigan, R.; Sampat, B.N. 2007. 'The Anatomy of Medical School Patenting'. *The New England journal of medicine* 357: 2049–2056.

Behrens, T.R. and Gray, D.O. 2001. 'Unintended consequences of cooperative research: Impact of industry sponsorship on climate for academic freedom and other graduate student outcome'. *Research Policy* 30: 179–199.

Bruneel, J.; D'Este, P.; Salter, A. 2010. 'Investigating the factors that diminish the barriers to university–industry collaboration'. *Research Policy* 39: 858–868.

de Chadarevian, S. 2011. 'The Making of an Entrepreneurial Science; Biotecknology in Britain, 1975–1995'. *Isis* 102: 601–633.

Chai, S. 2014. *Understanding Breakthrough Emergence through Missed Opportunities.* Working paper.

Cronin, B. and Sugimoto, C.R. 2014. *Beyond Bibliometrics : Harnessing Multidimensional Indicators of Scholarly Impact.* Cambridge: MIT Press.

Evans, J.A. 2010. 'Industry collaboration, scientific sharing, and the dissemination of knowledge'. *Social Studies of Science* 40: 757–791.

Folly, G.; Hajtman, B.; Nagy, J.I.; Ruff I. 1981. 'Some methodological problems in ranking scientists by citation analysis'. *Scientometrics* 3: 135–147.

Frängsmyr, T. 2008. 'Alfred Nobel'. *Swedish Institute:* 1–39.

Garfiled, E. 1970. 'Citation Indexing for Studying Science'. *Nature* 227: 669–671.

Garfield, E. and Malin, M.V. 1968. *Can Nobel Prize winners be predicted?* Paper presented at the 135th Annual Meeting of the American Association for the Advancement of Science, Dallas, Texas.

Gibbons, M. and Johnston, R. 1974. 'The roles of science in technological innovation'. *Research Policy* 3: 220–242.

Gingras, Y. and Wallace, M.L. 2010. 'Why it has become more difficult to predict Nobel Prize winners: a bibliometric analysis of nominees and winners of the chemistry and physics prizes (1901–2007)'. *Scientometrics* 82: 401–412.

Higgins, M.J.; Stephan, P.E.; Thursby, J.G. 2011. 'Conveying quality and value in emerging industries: Star scientists and the role of signals in biotechnology'. *Research Policy* 40: 605–617.

Johansson, J.E. 1926. 'Minneslista för Nobelprisgruppen Fysilogi och Medicin'. *Kungl. Boktryckeriet. P. A. Norstedt & Söner 253584.*

Larsson, U. 2008. 'Alfred Nobel: Networks of Innovations'. *Nobelmuseet, Gumanistika.*

Lindsten, J. and Ringertz, N. 2001. 'The Nobel Prize in Physiology or Medicine'. In *The Nobel Prizes:The First 100 Years*, edited by A. Wallin Levinovitz and N. Ringertz, 111–136. London: Imperial College Press and World Scientific Publishing Co. Pte. Ltd.

Link, A.N.; Siegel, D.S.; Bozeman, B. 2006. *An Empirical Analysis of the Propensity of Academics to Engage in Informal University Technology Transfer*, Troy.

Löfsten, H. and Lindelöf, P. 2005. 'R&D networks and product innovation patterns – Academic and non-academic new technology-based firms on Science Parks'. *Technovation* 25: 1025–1037.

Van Looy, B.; Callaert, J.; Debackere, K. 2006. 'Publication and patent behavior of academic researchers: Conflicting, reinforcing or merely co-existing?' *Research Policy* 35: 596–608.

Lundberg, J. et al. 2006. 'Collaboration uncovered: Exploring the adequacy of measuring university-industry collaboration through co-authorship and funding'. *Scientometrics* 69: 575–589.

Marks, LV. 2015. *The Lock and Key of Medicine: Monoclonal Antibodies and the Transformation of Healthcare.* New Haven: Yale University Press.

Merton, R.K. 1942. 'The Normative Structure of Science'. In *The Sociology of Science: Theoretical and Empirical Investigations*, edited by R.K. Merton, 267–278. Chicago: University of Chicago Press.

Merton, R.K. 1968. 'The Matthew Effect in Science'. *Science* 159: 56–63.

Mokyr, J. 2003. 'Thinking about Technology and Institutions'. *Macalester International* 13: 33–66.

Murray, F. 2004. 'The role of academic inventors in entrepreneurial firms: sharing the laboratory life'. *Research Policy* 33: 643–659.

Narin, F.; Pinski, G.; Gee, HH. 1976. 'Structure of the biomedical literature'. *J Am SOC Inform Sci* 27: 25–45.

National Science Board 2018. *Science and Engineering Indicators 2018.* Alexandria, VA: National Science Foundation (NSB-2018-1).

Nelson, R.R. 1996. *The Sources of Economic Growth.* London:Harvard University Press.

Nerkar, A. and Shane, S. 2003. 'When do start-ups that exploit patented academic knowledge survive?' *International Journal of Industrial Organization* 21: 1391–1410.

Nobelstiftelsens styrelse, 1925. 'Alfred Nobel och hans släkt'. *Almqvist & Wiksells boktryckeri-Aktiebolag.*

OECD. 2013. *Commercialising Public Research: New Trends and Strategies*, OECD Publishing. http://dx.doi.org/10.1787/9789264193321-en (accessed February 26, 2019).

Owen-Smith, J.; Riccaboni, M.; Pammolli, F.; Powell, W.W. 2002. 'A comparision of U.S and European University-Industry Relations in the Life Sciences'. *Management Science* 48: 24–43.

Perkmann, M. and Walsh, K. 2008. 'Engaging the scholar: Three types of academic consulting and their impact on universities and industry'. *Research Policy* 37: 1884–1891.

Perkmann, M.; King, Z.; Pavelin, S. 2011. 'Engaging excellence? Effects of faculty quality
on university engagement with industry'. *Research Policy* 40: 539–552.

Perkmann, M. et al. 2013. 'Academic engagement and commercialisation: A review of
the literature on university–industry relations'. *Research Policy* 42: 423–442.

Romer, P.M. 1990. 'Endogenous Technological Change.' *Journal of Political Economy* 98
(2): 71–102.

Slaughter, S. and Leslie, L.L. 2001. 'Expanding and Elaborating the Concept of Academic Capitalism'. *Organization* 8: 154–161.

De Solla Price, D.J. 1963. *Little science, big science.* New York: Columbia University Press.

Sorenson, O. and Fleming, L. 2004. 'Science and the diffusion of knowledge'. *Research
Policy* 33: 1615–1634.

Thomson, G. 2012. *Nobel Prizes that changed Medicine.* London: Imperial College Press
and World Scientific Publishing Co. Pte. Ltd.

Tushman, M. and Anderson, P. 1986. 'Technological Discontinuities and Organizational Environments'. *Administrative Science Quarterly* 31: 439–465.

Wuchty, S.; Jones, B.F.; Uzzi, B. 2007. 'Teams in Production of Knowledge.' *Science* 316:
1036–1040.

Zucker, L.G. and Darby, M.R. 1996. 'Star scientists and Institutional transformation: Patterns of invention and innovation in the formation of the biotechnology industry'.
Proc. Natl. Acad. Sci. USA 93: 12709–12716.

Zucker, L.G. and Darby, M.R. 2007. 'Virtuous circles in science and commerce'. *Pap. Reg.
Sci.* 86: 445–470.

Zucker, L.G.; Darby, M.R.; Armstrong, J.S. 2002. 'Commercializing Knowledge: University Science, Knowledge Capture, and Firm Performance in Biotechnology'. *Management Science* 48: 138–153.

Zuckerman, H. 1967. 'Nobel Laureates in Science: Patterns of Productivity, Collaboration, and Authorship'. *American Sociological Review* 32: 391–403.

Zuckerman, H. 1970. 'Stratification in American Science'. *Sociological Inquiry* 40:
235–257.

Zuckerman, H. 1977. *Scientific elite: Nobel laureates in the United States.* New Brunswick,
NJ: Transaction Publishers.

Index

Ackerknecht, Erwin   9
Adrian, Edgar D.   157, 165, 167
Afzelius, Ivar   48, 50
Agrawal, Ajay   195
Agre, Peter   175
Akerman, Jules   126
Alkarp, Magnus   72
Antoni, Nils   135
Arrhenius, Svante   44, 45, 48, 49, 49n, 50, 53,
   99, 101, 112, 117, 118, 118n
Arthus, Maurice   106
Asher, Leon   107
Auer, John   103, 106, 107
Avery, Oswald   30
Axelrod, Julius   167
Azoulay, Pierre   195

Bacq, Zénon M.   147
Baltimore, David   33, 178n
Banting, Frederick   123n
Bárány, Robert   123n
Barthes, Roland   143
Bartlett, John R.   33
Barton, Derek H.   192
Bataillon, Eugene   107, 114
Beck, Carl   126
Beck, Claude S.   128, 129n
Behring, Emil von   9, 19, 24, 83, 86–88, 99,
   103
Békésy, Georg von   158
Beneden, Édouard van   110
Bennett, Max R.   147
Berndt, Alfred   62, 63n
Bernhard, Carl G.   152, 153, 156, 156n, 161, 162
Bernheim, Alice   124
Bertrand, Albert   134
Bethe, Albrecht   105, 107
Bier, August   65, 115, 124
Billroth, Theodor   128, 128n
Binnig, Gerd   23
Bishop, Peter O.   154, 155, 155n, 161, 162
Björk, Ragnar   116
Black, James   28, 86, 177, 201
Blalock, Alfred   124, 128, 129, 136

Blumer, George   107
Bluntschli, Hans   107
Boberg, Ferdinand   43, 48
Bohr, Niels   53, 71
Boltzmann, Ludwig   101
Böök, Fredrik   61–65, 67, 68, 71–74
Borck, Cornelius   148, 169, 170
Bordet, Jules   59, 115
Borlaug, Norman   8ın
Bottazzi, Filippo   107
Bourdieu, Pierre   4, 35
Boveri, Theodor   110, 111
Bovet, Daniel   167
Boyd Orr, John   8ın
Boyle, Willard   17
Brachet, Albert   107
Brandt, Allan   89
Brannigan, Augustine   31
Branting, Fred   33
Branting, Hjalmar   48
Brock, Russel   128, 151
Brooks, Chandler McC.   150n
Brotherston, John H. F.   154
Brücke, Franz-Theodor von   152
Bucchi, Massimiano   117n, 161
Bud, Robert   85
Burnet, Frank McFarlane   85, 156
Butenandt, Adolf   67

Cajal, Santiago Ramon y   115, 166, 169
Campbell, William   86, 90
Carlsson, Gottfrid   65
Carrel, Alexis   27, 32, 33, 100, 103, 104, 107, 123,
   126, 127, 132, 133
Carrol, James   97
Carson, Rachel   29
Carter, H.   115
Casey, Brian P.   169
Casta, Laetitia   178–180, 182
Caullery, Maurice   107
Chain, Ernst   84
Cone, William   125
Cori, Carl   21
Cori, Gerty   21

Cormack, Allan M.   23
Cournand, André F.   22
Crafoord, Clarence   128
Cramér, Harald   88
Crawford, Elisabeth   19
Crick, Francis C.   23, 159
Croft, Simon   90, 91
Curie, Marie   33
Cushing, Harvey   124, 125, 133–136

Dale, Henry H.   10, 145, 147, 150, 158, 159,
     161–163, 166, 167, 169
Damadian, Raymond V.   30
Davidsson, David   51, 51n
De Sio, Fabio   98
DeBakey, Michael   130, 131, 131n
Delage, Yves   106, 113, 114
Dirac, Paul   53
Dogiel, Alexandre S.   107
Doherty, Peter   89
Dollinger, Julius   107
Domagk, Gerhard   28, 67, 70, 84
Dücker, Burckhard   6
Duffin, Jacalyn   34n, 83, 124, 162, 163
Dulbecco, Renato   10, 175, 177–186
Dunant, Henry   81n
Durkheim, Émile   35

Eccles, John C.   10, 98, 143–170
Edwards, Robert   26
Effler, Donald   130, 132
Ehrlich, Paul   23, 24, 83, 84, 87, 99, 101, 115,
     143
Eijkman, Christiaan   25, 115
Einthoven, Willem   22, 115, 136
Einstein, Albert   53, 71
Elion, Gertrude   28, 85, 201
Enders, John   89
Euler-Chelpin, Hans von   65–74
Euler-Chelpin, Ulf von   152, 159, 159n, 167
Ewald, Julius Richard   103, 105–109, 118

Farmer, Paul   81, 92
Fatt, Paul   149, 156
Favaloro, René   130–132
Fazio, Fabio   178–183, 186
Feldman, William   88

Felix, Wolfgang   108
Fenner, Frank   89
Fibiger, Johannes   24
Fick, Adolf   100
Fischer, Emil   11, 115
Fleck, Ludwik   3, 5, 21
Fleming, Alexander   84, 85, 123n
Flexner, Simon   103, 106, 107, 113, 117n
Finlay, Carlos J.   115
Flint, Joseph M.   107
Florey, Howard   84
Forbes, Alexander   150n
Forssmann, Werner   22, 123n
Fracastoro, Girolamo   24
Fracci, Carla   178
Franklin, Rosalind   23, 30
Franqué, O. von   107
Freeman, LM   129
Freud, Sigmund   30
Friedman, Robert M.   47, 135
Frisch, Karl von   29
Fulton, John F.   133
Funk, Casimir   25, 30

Gajdusek, D. Carleton   33
Galeotti, Gino   107
Galilei, Galileo   181, 181n
Garfield, Eugene E.   168n, 192
Garten, Siegfried   107
Gasser, Herbert S.   167
Gaule, Justus   103, 106, 107, 109, 110,
     111n
Gell-Mann, Murray   192
Gellhorn, Ernst   152, 160
Gellman, Jerome   35
Gérard, Pol   107
Gerard, Ralph W.   150n
Gibbon, John   128, 129
Gibson, William C.   169
Goebbels, Josef   71
Goetz, Robert   130–132
Goffman, Erving   3
Golgi, Camillo   22, 115, 167, 169
Goltz, Friedrich   100, 103, 105
Göring, Hermann   63, 67, 68, 73
Grafström, Sven   66, 73
Graham, Evarts   128

Granit, Ragnar   151–154, 157, 157n, 159–162, 167

Greene, Jeremy   89

Greyser, Stephen   39, 40

Grmek, Mirko   25

Gross, Robert   128

Grosz, Emile de   107, 111

Gullstrand, Allvar   22, 123n

Gurdon, John   192

Gütt, Arthur   66

Gutzmann, Hermann   115

Haber, Fritz   59

Hack, Margherita   185

Hahn, Otto   54

Halsted, William   124

Hamburger, Hartog J.   106

Hammarsten, Einar   55

Harrison, Ross G.   100, 114, 115

Hartline, Haldan K.   156, 157, 157n, 161

Hedin, Sven   65–68, 72, 72n

Heisenberg, Werner   53, 71

Helmholtz, Hermann von   102

Henderson, Rebecca   195

Henschen, Folke   67

Henschen, Salomon E.   51

Hertel, Ernst   107

Hertwig, Oscar   110–113

Hertwig, Richard   110, 112, 113, 114, 116

Hess, Walter R.   123n, 156

Hezel, Michael   203

Hinshaw, Corwin   88

Hippocrates   24, 33

Hitchings, George   28, 85, 201

Hitler, Adolf   8, 26, 60–63, 65–74

Hodgkin, Alan L.   144, 149, 149n, 151–154, 156–162, 167, 168

Hodgkin, Dorothy   23

Hoffmann, Paul   151, 160

Hofmeister, Franz   105, 107

Holmgren, Emil   109–111

Holmgren, Israel   67, 67n

Horsley, Victor   115, 124, 133, 133n, 134

Hounsfield, Godfrey N.   23

Hubel, David H.   167

Huggins, Charles   123n

Huisman, Frank   11

Humboldt, Alexander von   60

Huxley, Andrew F.   144, 149, 153, 154, 156–160, 162, 167

Ingram, Walter R.   134

Jacob, François   32

Johansson, Johan E.   49, 50, 51, 51n, 109, 113, 115, 116, 189, 193, 194

Jude, James R.   128, 129n

Jung, Richard   151

Kandel, Eric   32

Katz, Bernhard   145, 154, 156, 157, 167

Kaufmann, Jacob   108

Kendrew, John   23

Kim, Jim   92

Kitasato, Shibasaburo   30, 86

Knickerbocker, Guy   128, 129n

Koch, Robert   9, 19, 83, 85, 102

Kocher, Theodor   27, 115, 123, 124, 126, 133

Köhler, Georges   200

Kollesov, Vasili   130

Koranyi, Alexander   103, 103n, 106, 107, 112

Kouwenhoven, William B.   128, 129n

Krebs, Hans   21

Krönig, Bernhard   115

Kruif, Paul de   87n

Kuffler, Stephen W.   154

Kuhn, Richard   67

Kuhn, Thomas   21, 23

Laguesse, Edouard   108

Lammers, Hans H.   63n

Landsteiner, Karl   28

Lanz, Otto   125

Larsson, Ulf   203

Latour, Bruno   4, 5

Lauterbur, Paul C.   23

Laveran, Alphonse   115

Lawrence, Ernst   53, 54

Lederberg, Joshua   89, 90

Lenard, Philipp   71

Lennmalm, Frithiof   115, 134

Leriche, René   124

Lesch, John   84

Levene, Phoebus A.   103, 105–107, 113

Liebermann, Leo von   108
Liljestrand, Göran   50n, 54, 55, 98, 101, 104, 117
Lillehei, Walt   128
Lillie, Ralph S.   113, 114
Lind, James   25
Lindgren, Astrid   64
Lindhagen, Carl   51
Lindqvist, Sune   72
Lindsten, Jan   193, 194
Lippert, Justus   66
Lister, Joseph   123
Lloyd, David P. C.   146, 150, 150n, 156n
Loeb, Jacques   9, 10, 97–119
Loewi, Otto   167
Long, John H   108
Lorenz, Konrad   29
Lown, Bernard   81
Lubarsch, Otto   108
Lundborg, Herman   65
Luttenberger, Franz   48, 134

Mach, Ernst   100
Magee, Donald F.   159, 160
Magoun, Horace W.   156
Mall, Franklin P.   102, 107
Mansfield, Peter   23
Mao, Zedong   33
Marcus, Henry   135
Matthews, Albert P.   114
Marx, Karl   35
Maximow, Alexander A.   108
Maxwell, Samuel S.   110
Mayo, William   123
McCulloch, Warren S.   150n
McIntyre, Archibald K.   147n, 149n, 150n
Medawar, Peter B.   32, 156
Meitner, Lise   54
Meltzer, Samuel J.   105n, 106, 108
Mendel, Gregor   26
Merton, Robert K.   4, 31, 35, 97, 98, 143, 144n, 175, 176
Mesnil, Felix   107, 111
Meyer, Hans H.   108
Meyerhof, Otto   21, 119
Michelson, Albert A.   108, 111
Milstein, César   200
Minot, George   33

Moniz, António E.   27, 123, 133–136
Monod, Jacques   32
Montalcini, Rita L.   111, 112, 176, 178, 179, 183, 185
Moon, Sun Myung   165
Moore, Francis D.   122
Morgan, Thomas H.   26, 114
Mörner, Karl   83, 87, 88, 109, 111, 112, 112n, 113
Mühlhausen, Stefan   11
Müller, Erik   109, 113–115
Müller, Friedrich von   135
Müller, Paul   29
Münsterberg, Hugo   102, 105, 108, 118
Murphy, John B.   124, 136
Murray, Gordon   130
Murray, Joseph B.   28, 122, 123, 131

Nash, John   33
Natta, Giulio   177
Neuberg, Carl   116
Neurath, Constantin von   69
Nilsson-Ehle, Herman   65
Nó, Rafel Lorente de   150n
Nobel, Alfred   1, 10, 33, 40–42, 49, 52, 56, 60, 88, 102, 115, 125, 143, 178, 179, 188–191
Nobel, Emanuel   52
Nordin, Svante   61, 62, 63, 64
Norrby, Erling   89, 152n, 156, 158n, 159
Northrop, John H.   119

Ochsner, Albert J.   123
Odeberg, Hugo   65
Olivecrona, Karl   64, 65
Ōmura, Satoshi   86, 90
Orth, Johannes   110
Osborne, Oliver T.   108
Oseen, Carl Wilhelm   8
Ossietzky, Carl von   62, 68, 71, 72
Ostwald, Wilhelm   101, 117
Ostwald, Wolfgang   101, 103n
Overton, Ernest   109, 115

Palmquist, Åsa M.   203
Paulescu, Nicolai   30
Pauling, Linus   23
Pauly, Philip   100
Pavlov, Ivan P.   108, 111, 143
Payr, Erwin   124, 132

Penfield, Wilder 125, 133, 134, 136
Perutz, Max 23
Pfeiffer, Richard 8
Pfitzner, ? 110
Planck, Max 53, 60, 191
Popper, Karl R. 146–148, 150, 152, 163, 164, 164n, 166n
Porter, Michael 92
Prusiner, Stanley 89

Quincke, Heinrich I. 115

Rathenau, Walther 66
Rauber, August 108, 111
Ravi, Swati 203
Redelmeier, Robert J. 20, 34
Reed, Walter 97
Reverdin, Jacques L. 124
Richards, Alfred N. 108
Richards, Dickinson W. 22
Richet, Charles R. 102 , 106, 107, 117
Ringertz, Nils 193, 194
Ribbentrop, Joachim von 70
Robbins, Frederick C. 89, 167
Robinson, Edward G. 87n
Robson, Hugh N. 156, 157, 160, 161
Roentgen, Wilhelm Conrad 22
Rohrer, Heinrich 23
Rosenberg, Alfred 61, 65
Ross, Ronald 9
Roux, Émile 30, 83n, 99, 111
Roux, Wilhelm 101, 109, 110, 112
Ruska, Ernst 23
Rutherford, Ernest 101

Sabin, Albert 89
Sabin, Florence R. 108
Sabiston, David 130, 131
Salk, Jonas 88, 89
Sandler, Rickard 70n
Sartre, Jean-Paul 6
Sauerbruch, Ferdinand 65, 124
Schamberg, Jay F. 108
Schatz, Albert 30, 85n, 86
Schrödinger, Erwin 32, 53
Schultze, Bernhard 108
Schweitzer, Albert 81n
Sederholm, Henrik 49, 50

Senator, Hermann 108
Shakespeare, William 5
Shaw, Frank H. 147
Sherrington, Charles S. 10, 106, 119, 144–146, 150, 154, 155, 157, 160, 161, 164, 166–169
Siegbahn, Manne 53–55
Smith, Alexander 108, 111
Smith, Theobald 115
Söderqvist, Thomas 19
Sperry, Roger 32, 167
Standen, Anthony 32
Stark, Johannes 59, 71
Steinman, Ralph M. 19
Stewart, William H. 85n
Stieglitz, Julius 103, 106, 107, 111
Strahl, Hans 108
Strasburger, Eduard 110
Sundberg, Carl 115
Svartz, Nanna 84
Swain, Henry L. 108
Szentágothai, János 152

Tandler, Julius M. 107
Tangl, Franz 107, 111
Taussig, Helen B. 124, 128, 129, 136
Theorell, Hugo 55
Thomas, E. Donnall 28
Thucydides 24
Tinbergen, Nikolaas 29
Tiselius, Aarne 159
Tröhler, Ulrich 126

Udranszky, Ladislaus von 105, 107
Urde, Mats 39, 40

Verworn, Max 110
Virchow, Rudolf 22, 87, 102
Vries, Hugo de 101

Waksman, Selman 29, 30, 85, 85n, 86, 88
Wallenberg, Alice 54
Wallenberg, Knut 54
Warburg, Otto 21
Ward, Steven 90, 91
Wassermann, August von 107, 111, 113
Watson, James D. 23, 159
Weber, Max 35
Weinberg, Alvin 8

Weismann, August 111
Weismann, Friedrich 110
Weiss, Otto 108
Weller, Thomas 89
Whitley, Richard 3, 5
Whitteridge, David 154, 161
Widmalm, Sven 31n
Wied, Viktor zu 66, 68–70, 73, 73n
Wiesel, Torsten N. 167
Wilkins, Maurice H. F. 159
Winterstein, Hans 108

Wood, Stephanie 203
Wundt, Wilhelm 102

Yamanaka, Shinya 192
Youyou, Tu 86, 90

Zuckerman, Harriet 19, 176
Zuntz, Nathan 100, 101, 106, 108
Zunz, Edgard 108